Restoration
of the
Endodontically Treated Tooth

Herbert T. Shillingburg, Jr., D.D.S.
Professor and Chairman

James C. Kessler, B.S., D.D.S.
Assistant Professor

Department of Fixed Prosthodontics,
University of Oklahoma, College of Dentistry,
Oklahoma City, Oklahoma

Quintessence Publishing Co., Inc.   1982
Chicago, Berlin, Rio de Janeiro, Tokyo

Lithography: Industrie- und Presseklischee, Berlin; time litho, Leinfelden-Echterdingen
Composition and printing: F. W. Wesel, Baden-Baden
Binding: F. W. Wesel, Baden-Baden
Printed in Germany

ISBN 0-86715-108-0

Dedicated to

Connie

Peggy

Preface

Endodontic therapy in general, and the restoration of nonvital teeth in particular, fell into disrepute in the United States during the 1930's and 40's. The widespread disregard for prevention or elimination of infection in the restoration of pulpless teeth became linked with the medical profession's embrace of the *focus of infection* theory. Since the early 1950's, when endodontic therapy was put on a sound scientific footing, the restoration of nonvital teeth has once again increased in the United States.

The use of endodontic therapy has spread within the profession in this country, and its acceptance has grown within the patient population. This has created a new problem for dentistry. Teeth which would have been extracted at one time are now saved. Root canal therapy should not be considered as an end in itself, however: it is only the first phase of treatment. Not until the tooth has been restored to function consistent with the esthetic demands of the patient's mouth can the endodontic treatment be considered completed.

There are a number of dowel designs and techniques from which to choose in the restoration of the endodontically treated tooth. The last twenty years have seen a profusion of manufactured "systems" utilizing prefabricated dowels, and the literature has been filled with articles describing techniques for restoring the pulpless tooth. However, reports of controlled studies were rare before Colley's classic article on retention in 1968 and Standlee and Caputo's equally classic analysis of stress distribution in 1972. There have been many more research reports since that time. The group at U.C.L.A., with Dr. Jon Standlee and Dr. Angelo Caputo as its nucleus, continues to contribute objective data to this important clinical area.

In writing this book, we have attempted to focus on the underlying principles and the common aspects of the restoration of endodontically treated teeth, while presenting as many different techniques and systems as possible. Products in some classifications are *very* similar. There is often little to choose between in terms of real difference. The fact that one system was selected for a detailed technique description, while another was simply identified, does not imply an endorsement of one over the other. We hope that the similarities in product and technique will be evident. It is our hope that readers can use this book to become familiar with different ways of restoring endodontically treated teeth and to learn the actual techniques which seem attractive to them. Because new products and techniques are constantly being introduced, it is also hoped that this volume will help students of dentistry, whether undergraduate or practicing, to assess changes.

Acknowledgements

Our introduction to this subject in a rational, systematic manner can be traced to two fine dentists and teachers: Dr. Robert Dewhirst and Dr. Donald Fisher. Many of the principles articulated in this book were learned from them.

Ms. Julie Hall did her usual excellent job of typing, copying, and hieroglyphic interpretation. It is hard to imagine how the project would have progressed without her speed and accuracy.

Finally, the authors want to thank Dr. Randy Atkinson, Dr. Mark Felton, Dr. Ed Harroz, Dr. Robert Johnson, Dr. Neil White, Dr. Brad Williams, Dr. Ken Wilson, and Dr. Doug Woodson for their assistance with the clinical series.

Contents

Preface   7

Acknowledgements   9

Chapter 1   Principles of Restoration of Endodontically Treated Teeth   13

Chapter 2   Custom Dowel-Core (Direct)   45

Chapter 3   Custom Dowel-Core (Indirect)   75

Chapter 4   Custom Dowel-Core (Two-Piece)   95

Chapter 5   Dowel-Core Under a Crown   123

Chapter 6   Dowel-Inlay Crown Repair   143

Chapter 7   Precision Parallel Plastic Dowel   163

Chapter 8   Precision Tapered Plastic Dowel   181

Chapter 9   Prefabricated Dowel/Cast Core   205

Chapter 10   Prefabricated Dowel/Composite Resin Core   227

Chapter 11   Parallel Threaded Dowel (Pretapped)   253

Contents

Chapter 12   Parallel Self-Threading Dowel   275

Chapter 13   Tapered Self-Threading Dowel   291

Chapter 14   Amalgam Pin Core   313

Chapter 15   Composite Resin Pin Core   339

Chapter 16   Temporary Restorations for Endodontically Treated Teeth   357

Authors Index   375

Subject Index   379

Chapter 1

Principles of Restoration of Endodontically Treated Teeth

Restoration of the endodontically treated tooth is complicated by the fact that much or all of the coronal tooth structure which normally would be used in the retention of a restoration has been destroyed by caries, previous restorations, trauma, and the endodontic access preparation itself. The dentist must employ the principle of substitution, using a dowel in the root canal itself, or pins in the surrounding tooth structure, to build up a replacement for the missing coronal tooth structure. Only then can the tooth be restored.

Solutions to this problem have challenged the inventiveness and ingenuity of dentists for centuries. In fact, teeth were often intentionally devitalized so that the dentist could take advantage of the retention afforded by a dowel placed into the root canal. During the eighteenth century, Pierre Fauchard used a wooden post jammed into the canal to retain crowns. When the wood became wet, it swelled, making the fit even more snug and secure. It also, on occasion, split the root.

Early "pivot crowns" failed frequently because they were placed into poorly treated or totally untreated canals. The problem was such an obvious concern that one of the retentive devices, developed by Dr. F.H. Clark in 1849, consisted of a metal tube in the canal and a split metal dowel which was inserted into it.[1] This "spring-loaded" dowel was so designed to allow for the easy drainage of suppuration from within the canal or apical areas!

Even G.V. Black tackled this problem by developing a porcelain faced crown held in by a screw inserted into a canal filled with gold foil.[2] One design whose use persisted for a number of years was the Richmond crown. Introduced in 1880, it first consisted of a threaded tube in the canal which held a screw placed through the crown. This design was later simplified to eliminate the tube and make the dowel, by then unthreaded, an integral part of the final restoration or crown (Fig. 1-1).[3-6]

With the increased interest in the restoration of pulpless teeth in recent years,

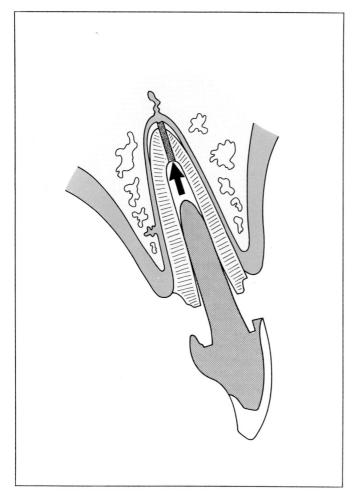

Fig. 1-1   At one time the dowel-crown, in which the dowel is an integral part of the crown, was a commonly used restoration design for restoring endodontically treated teeth. The Richmond crown is an example of this type.

there has been a gradual changeover from the crown in which the dowel is an integral part. In its place is a separate, well retained device which replaces the missing coronal tooth structure. The crown is fabricated over it as it would be fabricated over a preparation composed entirely of tooth structure (Fig. 1-2).

The supragingival portion of such a device, either because it replaces *coronal* tooth structure, or because it forms the center or core of the new restoration, or perhaps because of both, is referred to as a *core*. If it is retained by a dowel or post in the root canal, it is called a *dowel-core*. A third component of this system is an encircling band of metal which will support the tooth externally, bracing it against fracture by the dowel. This has been described as the "ferrule effect" by Eissmann, who suggests that it be 2.0 mm. wide.[7] It may be provided by a cop-

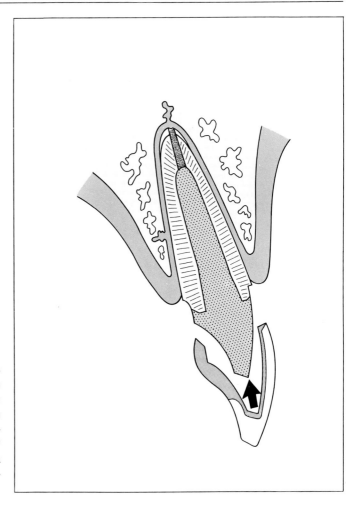

Fig. 1-2 The dowel-core utilizes a dowel in the root canal to retain the device, while the core portion replaces missing coronal tooth structure. The crown, a completely separate unit, is fabricated over the core as though it were a preparation in virgin tooth structure.

ing,[8] a long contrabevel on the core, or the axial walls of the crown, which extend apically beyond the margin of the dowel-core.

Finally, there must be a counter-rotational device on the dowel to prevent its being twisted or rotated by horizontal forces applied to the core. This can take the form of a keyway (a vertical groove cut in the wall of the canal, extending apically from the orifice),[9-16] an ovoid or irregularly shaped canal,[17-20] a short segment of a second root on a multi-rooted tooth,[21] or a pin hole parallel with and separate from the canal preparation.[22, 23] There is the possibility that the use of a keyway could endanger the structural integrity of the root.[24] If a deep keyway is placed in a thin-walled tooth, it could act as a wedge and produce a cleavage plane. A keyway of normal depth and length placed in an adequate bulk of tooth structure is not likely to have a deleterious effect, however.

If the core is retained by small pins placed in the dentin around the root canal, it is a *pin-retained core.* Components may be prefabricated or custom-made, and they can be combined with cast metals or plastic material placed in the mouth. In any event, all devices used for building up teeth are variations of the dowel-core or the pin-retained core.

There are distinct advantages in having the retention device separate from the crown restoring the tooth. The adaptation of the axial walls and margin of the crown are totally unrelated to the fit of the dowel in the canal. Secondly, the crown can be easily remade if that should become necessary because of materials failure, caries, or change in the role of the crown (from simple restoration to bridge retainer) at anytime in the future. Replacing a single piece dowel-crown can be most difficult if the dowel is of adequate length. Although devices have been described for removing crowns, the force required to remove a crown with a long dowel just about dictates the cutting of a crown preparation in solid porcelain and metal (Fig. 1-3a and b). If it can be done, it will be time-consuming and tiring for both dentist and patient. Finally, if the tooth being restored is to be used as a bridge abutment, it is not necessary to attempt to align the canal preparation with the path of insertion of the other abutment preparation(s), or vice versa.

The decision of whether to use some form of dowel-core or a pin-retained core is dependent upon several inter-related factors: the thickness of tooth structure around the canal, the bulk and height of remaining supragingival tooth structure, the diameter of the tooth, root morphology, bone support, and the tooth's role in the final restoration of the mouth (single restoration or abutment).

Not every endodontically treated tooth will require a crown. If an anterior tooth has sustained only minimal damage in the past, with no proximal surface involvement, it may be possible to restore the tooth with a lingual composite. Such a circumstance is the exception, however, and more extensive restoration is generally required. It is recommended by several authors that no less be done for an endodontically treated tooth than the placement of a restoration which will provide occlusal coverage.[25–30]

For those teeth that will require a crown, a decision must be made regarding the type of core required. Numerous clinicians have held that the tooth should be reinforced with a dowel.[7, 16, 20, 31–36] Laboratory studies of the subject have been only partially supportive. Guzy and Nicholls, applying forces at 130° to the long axis, found no difference in the failure loads of canines or incisors which were reinforced with 1.0 mm. diameter posts compared with those which were unprotected.[37] Kantor and Pines, however, reported that teeth with 1.25 mm. posts were 56% stronger than control teeth upon which no endodontic procedure had been performed, with loads applied at a 45° angle.[38] Trabert and associates, using an impact tester, discovered no difference in resistance to fracture between untreated control teeth

Fig. 1-3 Considerable difficulty may be encountered when a dowel-crown, such as the one on this maxillary right central incisor, must be replaced (a). If the original dowel was of adequate length, the dentist may have to create a preparation for the next crown from solid metal in the mouth (b).

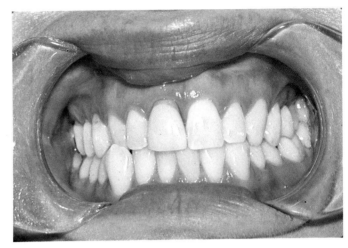

Figure 1-3a

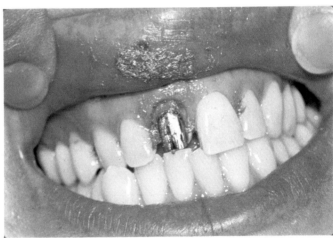

Figure 1-3b

and endodontically treated teeth without posts.[39] When teeth were restored with a steel post 1.25 mm. in diameter, however, the teeth were less likely to fracture than either the controls or teeth "reinforced" with a larger 1.75 mm. post.

There would seem to be some basis for placing a dowel in the anterior tooth whose small root cross section does not possess the necessary bulk to provide adequate protection from fracture fol-lowing the endodontic treatment. The dowel must not be made so large, however, that it destroys valuable tooth structure, and with it the structural integrity and natural strength of the tooth. The large circumference of a posterior tooth eliminates the need for a dowel to reinforce the tooth.[7] Dowels may be used in posterior teeth to improve retention and to support the core and crown against laterally directed forces when

17

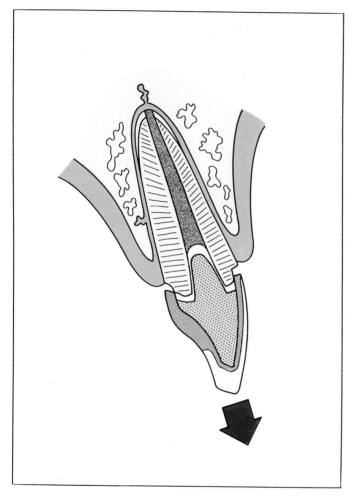

Fig. 1-4 Short dowels offer little resistance to displacement from either axially or obliquely directed forces.

there is no remaining coronal tooth structure to serve that function.

Dowel Retention

There are four factors which can have an effect on the retention of any dowel: length, taper, diameter, and surface configuration.

Dowel Length. It is not surprising that length plays the same role in the retention of dowel-cores that it does in the retention of crowns:/i.e., as length increases, so does retention. Inadequate length in dowels is probably the leading cause of failure of restorations on endodontically treated teeth (Fig. 1-4). Colley and associates demonstrated 2.23 times as much retention by increasing dowel length from 5.5 mm. to 8.0

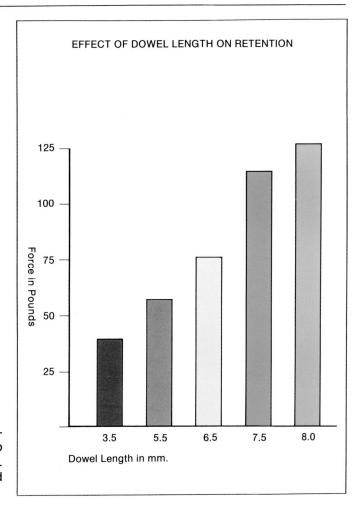

EFFECT OF DOWEL LENGTH ON RETENTION

Force in Pounds

125 —

100 —

75 —

50 —

25 —

3.5   5.5   6.5   7.5   8.0

Dowel Length in mm.

Fig. 1-5 This graph demonstrates the direct relationship between length and retention. (Based on data by Colley and associates.[40])

mm. (Fig. 1-5).[40] Other studies have reinforced this finding. Krupp et al. found an average increase of 47% in retention for an increase from 5.0 to 8.0 mm.[41] An increase in retention of approximately 43% was shown by Johnson and Sakumura when the dowel was lengthened from 7.0 to 11.0 mm.[42] Standlee et al. showed that the retention for all types of dowels was about one and one-half times as great when embedment depth increased from 5.0 to 8.0 mm.[43] Ruemping and associates also determined that tensile retention increased with length, but they found that it was only 1.23 times as great when the dowel was expanded from 5.0 to 8.0 mm.[14]

Because of its great importance to the longevity of the restoration, dowel length has attracted the attention of numerous clinicians writing on the subject. Many authors feel that the minimum length of

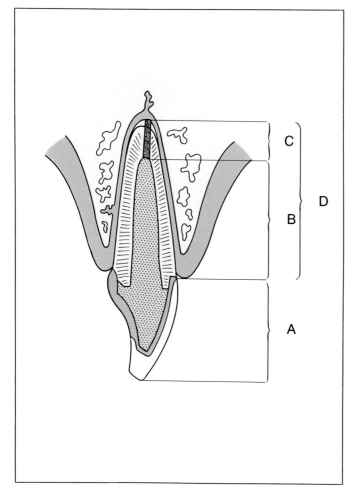

Fig. 1-6 To provide maximum retention, the dowel should equal the crown in length (A = B), or be two-thirds the length of the root (B = D), whichever is greater. The length of gutta percha remaining at the apex (C) should be a minimum of 4.0 mm.

the dowel should be equal to the length of the crown.[3, 4, 9, 13, 16, 19–21, 28–30, 44–61] Others have stated that the dowel should be two-thirds the length of the root.[7, 10, 11, 20, 29, 44, 51, 52, 62–71] A dowel length equal to three-quarters of the root length has been projected as the ideal by a few authors.[11, 62, 63, 72] Other dowel lengths which have been proposed include half the length of the canal,[57, 73, 74] 80% of the root,[75] 133% of the crown,[12] 150% of the crown,[76] and, in techniques in which the dowel doubles as the root canal filling, equal to the length of the root.[77, 78]

Another dimension relating to dowel-cores which must be considered is the length of root canal filling left at the apex (Fig. 1-6). The minimum length of the remaining apical fill has been set variously at 3.0 mm.,[13, 21, 47, 58, 79] 3-5 mm.,[49, 76] 4.0 mm.,[80] and 4-5 mm.[36] As the apex is approached, the possibility of dislodging

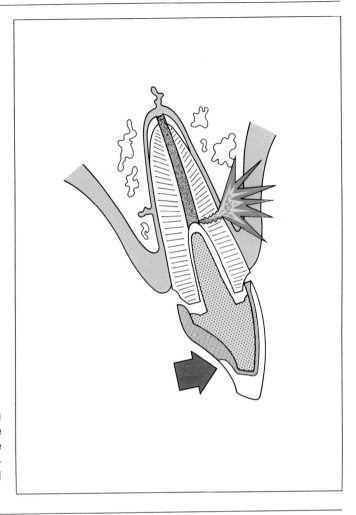

Fig. 1-7   In addition to exhibiting poor retention, short dowels are more likely to cause root fracture from stresses generated by occlusal forces on the crown and dowel-core.

the root canal filling increases. There is also the possibility that an unfilled accessory or lateral canal will be uncovered, causing an infection of periapical tissues. The optimum distance between the end of the dowel and the apex is 4.0 mm., with a greater length left when a longer root length will permit it. Besides providing poor retention, a short dowel can also lead to fracture of the root. [58, 69] If the end of the dowel is at or above the alveolar crest of bone, that part of the root investing the dowel will not be bolstered by bone against forces transmitted from the dowel to the tooth. Occlusal forces can produce stresses in the unsupported root, fracturing it diagonally from the tip of the dowel down to the crest of bone[17] (Fig. 1-7). For that reason, some authors have suggested that the dowel be embedded far enough into the root so that it will extend at least

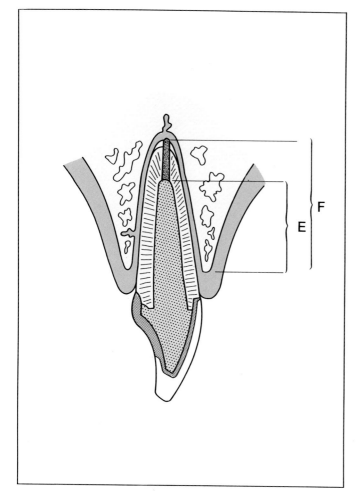

Fig. 1-8   To protect the root from fracture, the length of dowel from alveolar crest to apical end should be at least half the length of the root embedded in bone (E = ½ F).

one-half the distance from the alveolar crest to the apex of the root (Fig. 1-8).[15, 17, 35, 81, 82]

Kurer estimates that it is not possible to achieve a dowel equal in length to the crown in 20-25% of the cases.[83] A quick comparison of crown and root lengths indicates that this assumption is anatomically correct (Table 1-1), although the clinical crown would be slightly shorter. A dowel equal in length to the crown would encroach on the 4.0 mm. apical safety zone in the average maxillary or mandibular incisor.

What then should be the length of the dowel? Simply stated, it should be as long as possible.[51] A dowel length equal to that of the crown, or to two-thirds that of the root, is a good rule of thumb. Comparison of the crown and root lengths becomes especially significant when all coronal tooth structure has been de-

TABLE 1-1   **Crown and Root Lengths (in mm.)**[84]

	Average Crown Length	Average Root Length			2/3 Root Length			4 mm. from Apex		
Maxillary Teeth										
Central Incisor	10.8	12.5			8.3			8.5		
Lateral Incisor	9.7	13.1			8.7			9.1		
Canine	10.2	15.8			10.5			11.8		
First Premolar	8.6	12.7			8.5			8.7		
Second Premolar	7.5	13.5			9.0			9.5		
		MF	DF	L	MF	DF	L	MF	DF	L
First Molar	7.4	12.5	12.0	13.2	8.3	8.0	8.8	8.5	8.0	9.2
Second Molar	7.4	12.8	12.0	13.4	8.5	8.0	8.9	8.8	8.0	9.4
Madibular Teeth										
Central Incisor	9.1	12.4			8.3			8.4		
Lateral Incisor	9.4	13.0			8.7			9.0		
Canine	10.9	14.3			9.5			10.3		
First Premolar	8.7	13.4			8.9			9.4		
Second Premolar	7.8	13.6			9.1			9.6		
		M	D		M	D		M	D	
First Molar	7.4	13.5	13.4		9.0	8.9		9.5	9.4	
Second Molar	7.5	13.4	13.3		8.9	8.9		9.4	9.3	

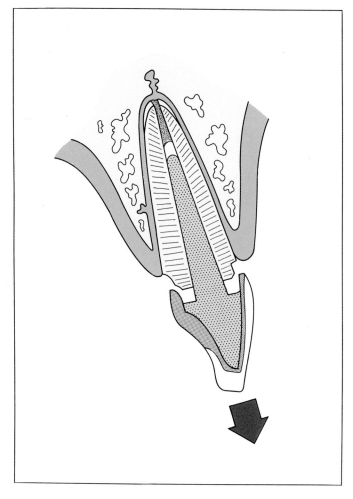

Fig. 1-9 Tapered dowels are not as retentive as parallel-sided ones.

stroyed. If intact coronal tooth structure is preserved, as many clinicians recommend,[12, 15, 34, 44, 45, 54, 63, 82, 85–87] the dowel length is measured from the occlusal end of that intact coronal tooth structure. It is not necessary under those conditions to extend as far apically to achieve a given dowel length.

Dowel Taper. The taper of the walls of a dowel has a direct bearing on the be-

havior of the dowel in the tooth. Parallel-sided dowels are more retentive than tapered dowels (Fig. 1-9). In various studies, this superiority in retention has been demonstrated to be 1.9 times,[40] 3.3 times,[43] and 4.5 times[42] as great as that of the tapered dowels. The tapered dowel also generates greater stress than does the parallel dowel,[23, 85] showing a potential for splitting the root[88] (Fig. 1-10). The tapered dowel tends to produce greater

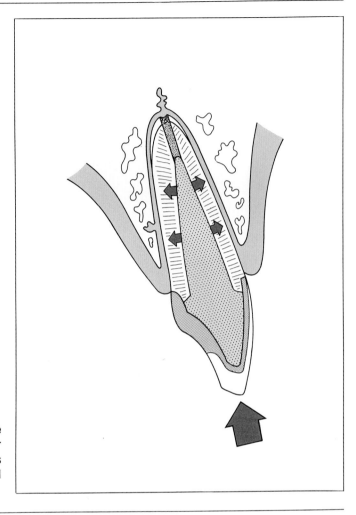

Fig. 1-10 Tapered dowels are capable of generating greater stress in the root around them, as occlusal forces are transmitted outward in a wedge-like fashion.

stress in the shoulder area of the restoration, while the parallel-sided dowel causes more stress in the apical area, especially during cementation.[89] In an effort to minimize the splitting potential of a tapered dowel, there should be a flat seat at the occlusal end of the preparation to resist apically directed forces and prevent wedging.[13, 17, 35]

The proximity of the edge of a parallel dowel to the periphery of a tapered root also could increase the danger of a lateral perforation. This has led some dentists to opt for the less retentive tapered dowel to avoid a possible apical perforation or fracture.[40, 51] This is more of a concern in teeth whose roots are thin and fragile.

Dowel Diameter. The diameter of a dowel has an effect on both the retention of the restoration and its strength and ability to

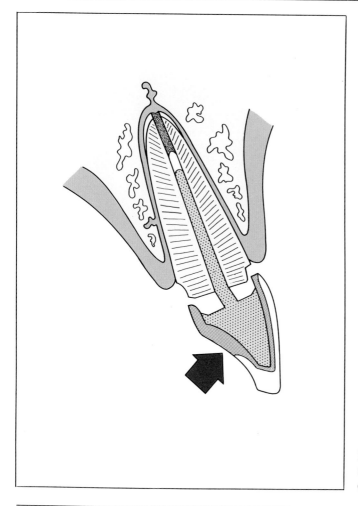

Fig. 1-11 Thin dowels are less retentive and more easily distorted by occlusal forces.

resist distortion. The smaller the diameter of a dowel, the more likely that it will be displaced, with or without accompanying distortion or fracture (Fig. 1-11). Increasing the diameter of 5.0 mm. long parallel dowels by 0.25 mm. increased retention by 53% in one study[41] and by 47% in another,[90] while enlarging the diameter of a 7.0 mm. long parallel dowel by 0.35 mm. produced a 45% increase in a third investigation.[42] Although it is unquestionably effective, enlarging the

dowel is not the safest way of improving retention because it does destroy and weaken the remaining tooth.[23] At best, the enlarged dowel does not contribute to the strength of the tooth.[39] At worst, it could cause a fracture and loss of the tooth (Fig. 1-12).

One-third the diameter of the root has been proposed as a clinical guideline for the width of the dowel.[34, 82] It has also been suggested that there be 1.0 mm. between the wall of the prepared canal

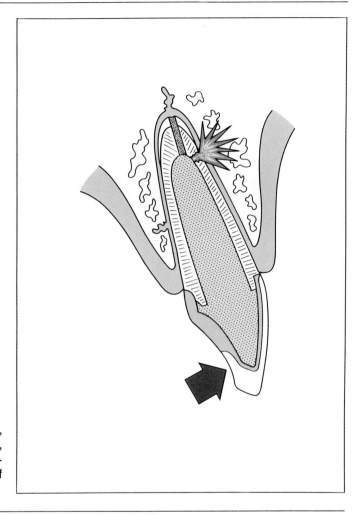

Fig. 1-12 Oversized dowels, which are strong in themselves, achieve that strength at the expense of the structural integrity of the root.

and the outer surface of the root.[23] The diameter of the dowel will be determined, to some extent, by the narrowest portion of the root. This will be the mesiodistal width of most roots, measured 4.0 mm. from the apex. The thickness of tooth structure in this area is important as a safeguard against perforation of the root.

Because of the faciolingual direction of much occlusal force, the amount of tooth structure between the dowel and the outer surface of the root on the facial and lingual aspects of the root is quite important in protecting the structural integrity of the root. Most roots exhibit considerably thicker dentin faciolingually than they do mesiodistally.

Therefore, a dowel whose diameter is less than one-third the faciolingual dimension of the root at the midpoint of the dowel may be large enough to exceed one-third of the mesiodistal width of the root. This can still be acceptable if the dowel is small enough not to encroach on the mesial and distal surfaces of the root. To this end, the mesiodistal diameter of a dowel should be 2.0 mm. less than that of the root at the midpoint of the dowel and 1.5 mm. less than that of the root at the dowel's end. Root dimensions and recommended dowel widths are shown for maxillary teeth in Table 1-2, while those for mandibular teeth can be found in Table 1-3. Because of the factors mentioned above, they are slightly larger than those recommended in a previous study.[91]

These dimensions should be used only for determining the size of dowel that normally would be used. It is just as important to measure the width of a root as it is to assess its length when judging the size of dowel that will be placed in a tooth.

Dowel Surface. Dowels can be categorized in several ways. Classification can be made by their geometric shape–tapered or parallel–and by their surface configuration–smooth, serrated, or threaded (Fig. 1-13). Surface configuration probably plays the single most important role in retention. Threaded dowels are unquestionably the most retentive. Standlee and associates found the pretapped, parallel-sided, threaded dowel to be twice as retentive as a parallel-sided serrated dowel and approximately 6.6 times as retentive as a smooth-sided tapered dowel[43] (Fig. 1-14). Ruemping et al. found it 5 and 7 times as retentive, respectively.[14]

The use of threaded dowels is accompanied by some controversy, however.

They do generate greater stresses than do other types of dowels.[71, 85, 89] The tapered threaded dowel presents a particular hazard because of the combination of a taper and threads. There is some feeling that to be used successfully it should be passively inserted as a modified cemented dowel.[23, 30] A study on root fractures showed that the torque required to insert tapered threaded dowels was approximately 25% of that required to fracture a root.[92] The tap for a parallel threaded dowel was not able to effect a root fracture in the same study. The stresses[89] and the forces[92] generated by tapping the root canal can be minimized by frequently cleaning the tap during the process. These studies, of course, do not assess the effect, if any, of the threaded anchor functioning under occlusal loads for a prolonged period of time. They should be used with caution.

Dowels with serrated walls which do not actively engage the sides of the canal are more retentive than the smooth-surfaced dowel. Colley and associates found serrated parallel posts to be 4.3 times as retentive as their smooth counterparts.[40] The effect of taper on retention has already been discussed.

Cementation

There are several types of cements which can be used for the placement of dowels in the canal. One study on the retention of dowels by different cements has shown a slight superiority of zinc phosphate over polycarboxylate and epoxy cements when used with tapered

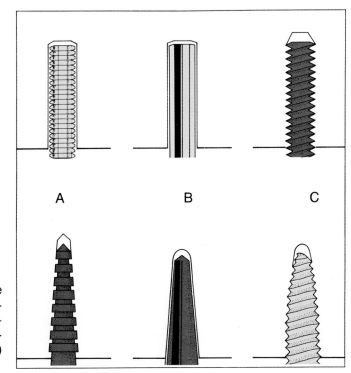

Fig. 1-13 All dowels can be classified by geometry: parallel-sided (top row) or tapered (bottom row); and by surface configuration: (A) serrated, (B) smooth, (C) threaded.

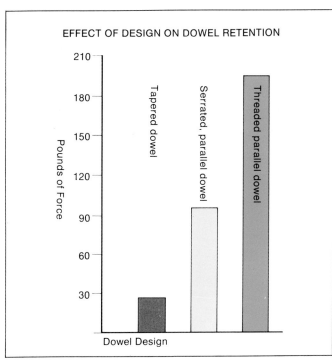

EFFECT OF DESIGN ON DOWEL RETENTION

Fig. 1-14 This graph shows the difference in retention produced by surface configuration. (Based on data by Standlee et al.[43])

TABLE 1-2 **Root Diameter and Dowel Size for Maxillary Teeth (in mm.)**[84]

		CEJ	Midpoint*	4 mm. from Apex**	Dowel Size
Central Incisor	M-D	6.3	5.2	3.8	1.7
	F-L	6.4	5.8	4.3	
Lateral Incisor	M-D	4.9	4.0	3.2	1.3
	F-L	5.7	5.4	4.2	
Canine	M-D	5.4	4.4	3.3	1.5
	F-L	7.7	7.2	4.8	
First Premolar	M-D	4.1	Facial M-D 3.6	2.6	0.9
	F-L	8.1	F-L 3.4	2.4	
			Lingual M-D 3.3	2.5	0.9
			F-L 3.3	2.4	
Second Premolar	M-D	4.9	3.8	3.2	1.1
	F-L	7.9	7.0	5.0	
First Molar	M-D	7.7	Mesio- M-D 3.4	2.9	1.1
	F-L	10.5	facial F-L 6.8	4.8	
			Disto- M-D 3.1	2.6	1.1
			facial F-L 5.0	3.8	
			Lingual M-D 5.7	4.4	1.3
			F-L 4.3	3.3	
Second Molar	M-D	7.3	Mesio- M-D 3.4	2.7	1.1
	F-L	10.4	facial F-L 6.6	4.5	
			Disto- M-D 3.1	2.4	0.9
			facial F-L 4.3	3.2	
			Lingual M-D 4.9	3.6	1.3
			F-L 4.5	3.1	

* On the first and second molars the middle measurement was made at the furcation, which is 4.1 mm. from the cemento-enamel junction on the first molar, and 3.2 mm. on the second molar.

** Because of greater root length, the mean distance from the apex on canine measurements was 5.1 mm.

TABLE 1-3   Root Diameter and Dowel Size for Mandibular Teeth (in mm.) [84]

		CEJ	Midpoint*	4 mm. from Apex	Dowel Size
Central Incisor	M-D	3.3	2.7	2.1	0.7
	F-L	5.5	5.6	4.3	
Lateral Incisor	M-D	3.6	2.7	2.0	0.7
	F-L	5.9	5.7	4.3	
Canine	M-D	5.2	4.0	3.2	1.5
	F-L	7.8	7.3	5.0	
First Premolar	M-D	5.1	4.0	3.2	1.3
	F-L	6.6	6.0	4.3	
Second Premolar	M-D	5.3	4.3	3.5	1.3
	F-L	7.0	6.0	4.4	
First Molar	M-D	8.9	Mesio- M-D 3.7	2.8	1.1
	F-L	8.3	facial F-L 3.4	2.8	
			Mesio- M-D 3.4	2.5	0.9
			lingual F-L 3.5	2.7	
			Distal M-D 3.5	2.7	1.1
			F-L 7.6	5.4	
Second Molar	M-D	9.3	Mesio- M-D 3.6	2.6	0.9
	F-L	8.3	facial F-L 3.2	2.4	
			Mesio- M-D 3.6	2.5	0.9
			lingual F-L 3.2	2.3	
			Distal M-D 4.1	3.0	1.1
			F-L 6.8	4.7	

* On the first and second molars the middle measurement was made at the furcation, which is 3.1 mm. from the cemento-enamel junction on the first molar, and 3.3 mm. on the second molar.

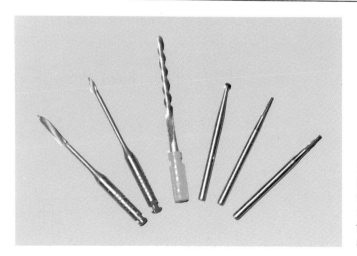

Fig. 1-15 Some of the types of instruments used for instrumenting the dowel space, from left to right: safe-ended reamers, hand file, standard burs with long shanks.

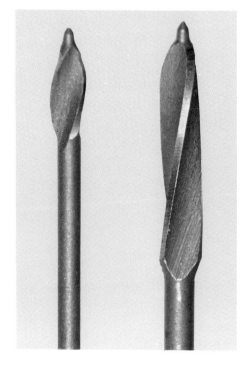

Fig. 1-16 The Gates Glidden drill (left) shares several common traits with the Peeso reamer (right): a non-cutting tip and a similar configuration in the cutting end. On the other hand, the Gates Glidden drill has much shorter cutting flutes (1.5–4.0 mm.) than those of the Peeso reamer (7.5–8.5 mm.). All sizes of both instruments measure 18 mm. from the cutting end (*base* of the safety tip) to the end of the tapered shaft, which is flush with the head of the handpiece.

dowels.[43] In the same study by Standlee et al., there were no differences among the cements when used with other dowel designs.

Hanson and Caputo found no significant long-term differences among polycarboxylate, zinc phosphate, and ethyl cyano-acrylate cements with parallel serrated dowels, although the cyano-acrylate was most retentive 1.5 hours after cementation.[90] A third study from the same group showed that the newer glass ionomer cements offered no advantage over other types of cements for dowel retention.[41] Neither medication with camphorated parachlorophenol nor pretreatment with citric acid produced any significant difference.

It is important that the dowel to be cemented have a vent on its side to relieve hydrostatic back pressure.[89] This may be in the form of a v-shaped groove[11, 51] or a flat side on the round dowel.[71]

Instrumentation

A wide variety of instruments can be used for enlarging the root canal for a dowel (Fig. 1-15), ranging from standard burs with elongated shanks to endodontic hand reamers to special safe-ended handpiece reamers made for the purpose. Preparation of the dowel space would best be done at the time of the endodontic procedure, simply because the dentist who performs the root canal obturation will be most familiar with the morphology and topographical features of the canal.[93] However, there appears to be no significant advantage in protecting the apical seal by enlarging the canal

soon after completion of endodontic therapy. Neagley found little leakage around laterally condensed gutta percha points when they were prepared for dowel spaces using burs and Peeso reamers.[94] In that same study, however, 89% of the silver points which were shortened by 1.0 mm. during dowel space preparation showed leakage. No leakage was seen if the burs or reamers were stopped short of touching the silver points.

Restorations for endodontically treated teeth are most easily and safely done in teeth treated with gutta percha. Teeth treated with silver points can be restored *if* the silver points are prenotched and twisted off at the time of placement.[47, 94–98] If the silver point is touched by a rotary instrument during the preparation, the apical seal will be broken. If a full length silver point is present in the tooth, it should be retrieved and the tooth retreated with gutta percha.

The preparation is begun by placing a hot endodontic plugger approximately half the length of the canal. This is followed by the actual dowel preparation. Peeso reamers or Gates Glidden drills are widely used for preparing the dowel space (Fig. 1-16).[9, 11, 13, 16, 47, 50, 51, 54, 71, 86, 99, 100] Because they have a sharp, but noncutting, tip, they will follow the path of least resistance, which is the cleared canal or the gutta percha in the canal (Fig. 1-17). Peeso reamers will also conform more consistently to the original canal in the apical region than will other types of instruments.[101]

Begin with the largest size that will fit easily into the canal. Prepare the canal to

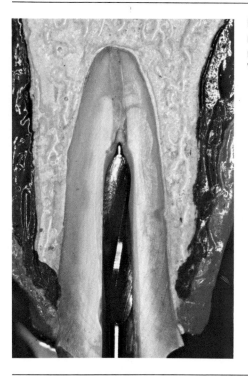

Fig. 1-17 The sharp non-cutting tip of the Peeso reamer follows the path of least resistance: the root canal. (Photograph courtesy of Dr. Donald W. Fisher).

the complete predetermined length. Then switch to the next largest instrument in the graduated series and repeat the process. Do this until the desired diameter has been attained. Gates Glidden drills are easily used because the cutting portion is smaller and more maneuverable. They are often easier to use in starting very small canals (Fig. 1-18a). The preparation should be completed with the series of Peeso reamers, however (Fig. 1-18b). The longer cutting segment in it will prepare a straighter canal wall with less liklihood of an undercut. The instrument is leaned over slightly as it is withdrawn from the mouth of the canal. This will result in an essentially parallel-sided preparation with a tapered orifice.

Standard burs can also be used for making the dowel preparation (Fig. 1-19). Both round burs[12, 19, 32, 45, 102, 103] and tapered fissure burs[3, 88, 103] have been recommended for this purpose. In the hands of an inexperienced operator, these instruments can more easily go astray. This is a particular hazard if the bur is much larger than the cleared canal, or if the bur is extended to a level from which the gutta percha has not been removed.

Custom vs. Prefabricated

A custom dowel-core can be made by relining a plastic sprue with acrylic, or a metal pin with wax, to form the dowel.

Fig. 1-18 The Peeso reamers (a), numbered 1-6, range in diameter from 0.7 to 1.7 mm. in graduated increments of 0.2 mm. The Gates Glidden drills (b), distinguished by their shorter cutting flutes and more flexible shafts, use the same numbering system. The sizes range from 0.6 to 1.5 mm., however, so that a No. 4 Peeso reamer (1.3 mm.) and a No. 4 Gates Glidden drill (1.1 mm.) are *not* the same diameter.

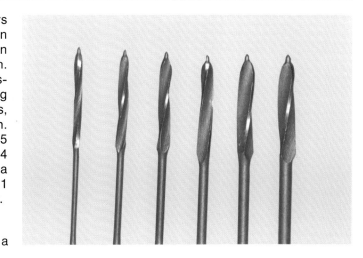

a

b

Fig. 1-19 The standard burs which are used by some dentists for enlarging the dowel space include (from left to right) the No. 4 round bur, the No. 700 tapered fissure bur and the No. 701 tapered fissure bur.

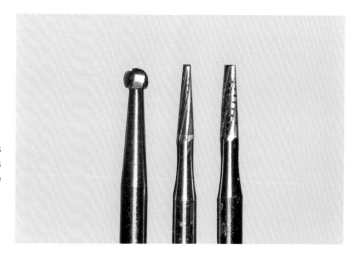

35

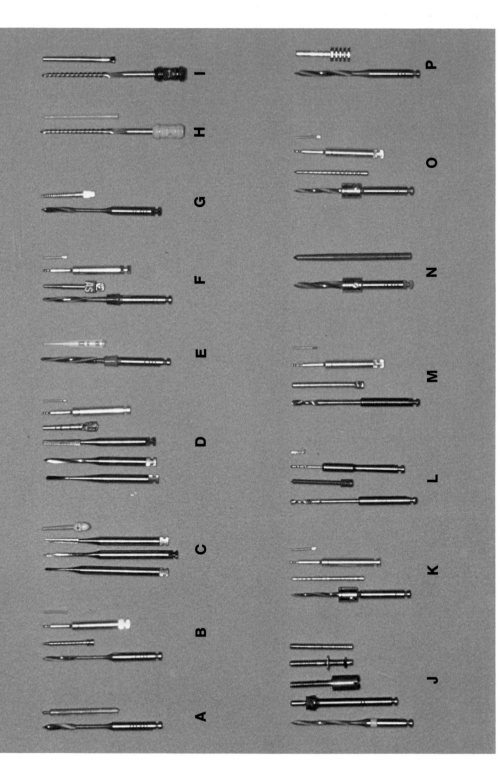

Fig. 1-20 Instruments and dowels of commonly used dowel systems are shown above:

A. Peeso reamer
    Solid plastic sprue

    Union Broach Corp.
    Williams Gold
    Refining Co.

B. Peeso reamer BCH Post
    0.5 mm. Kodex drill &
    Minim pin

    Unitek Corp.
    Whaledent
    International

C. Calibrated Instrument burs
    Resin dowel

    Parkell

D. Calibrated Instrument burs
    Steel dowel
    0.5 mm. Kodex drill &
    Minim pin

    Parkell

    Whaledent
    International

E. Colorama reamer
    Plastic dowel

    J. Aderer, Inc.

F. Colorama reamer
    Steel dowel
    0.5 mm. Kodex drill &
    Minim pin

    J. Aderer, Inc.

    Whaledent
    International

G. Peeso reamer
    Dentatus Screw Post

    Union Broach Corp.

H. Hand file
    Endowel plastic dowel

    Star Dental Manufac-
    turing Co.

I. Hand file
    Endo-Post metal dowel

    Kerr Dental Manufac-
    turing Co.

J. Kurer reamer and root
    facer
    Crown Anchor
    Fin-lock Anchor
    Crown Saver

    Teledyne Getz

K. NuBond Fast Post reamer
    Stainless steel Fast Post
    0.5 mm. Kodex drill &
    Minim pin

    Ellman International
    Mfg.
    Whaledent
    International

L. Para-Post drill
    Para-Post plastic dowel
    0.7 mm. Paramax drill &
    iridio-platinum pin

    Whaledent
    International

M. Para-Post drill
    Para-Post steel dowel
    0.5 mm. Kodex drill &
    Minim pin

    Whaledent
    International

N. P-D reamer/
    P-D acrylic dowel

    Union Broach Corp.

O. P-D reamer
    P-D stainless steel crown
    post
    0.5 mm. Kodex drill &
    Minim pin

    Union Broach Corp.

P. Radix reamer
    Radix anchor

    Star Dental Manufac-
    turing Co.

TABLE 1-4 Specifications of Dowels and Reamers

DIAMETER (in mm.)

DOWEL	TAPER	TYPE	SURFACE	Specifications across diameter (0.5–2.4 mm)
BCH	0°	Stainless Steel Dowel	Serrated	2– 8 Post, 2–10 Post; 3– 8 Post, 3–10 Post, 3–12 Post; 4–10 Post, 4–12 Post, 4–14 Post; 5–12 Post, 5–14 Post, 5–16 Post; 6–16 Post, 6–18 Post, 6–20 Post
		Precision Plastic Pattern	Smooth	
C · I	2.6°	Stainless Steel Dowel	Serrated	Small Bibevel Twist Drill "A"; Small Reamer "B"; Small Bur "C"; Small Resin Post; Small Steel Post; Medium Bibevel Twist Drill "A"; Medium Reamer "B"; Medium Bur "C"; Medium Resin Post; Medium Steel Post
Colorama	0°/ 6.2°	Precision Plastic Pattern	Smooth	A11 (yellow) Reamer & Posts; A12 (red) Reamer & Posts; A13 (blue) Reamer & Posts; A14 (green) Reamer(s) & Posts; A15 (black) Reamer(s) & Posts
		Stainless Steel Dowel	Smooth	
Dentatus	Var.	Self-Threading Gold Plated Brass Dowel	Threaded	No. 1 Short/Med/Long; No. 2 Short/Med/Long; No. 3 Short/Med/Long; No. 4 Short/Med/Long Ex Long; No. 5 Short/Med/Long Ex Long; No. 6 Short/Med/Long Ex Long
Endowel	1.1°	Precision Plastic Pattern	Smooth	No. 70, No. 80, No. 90, No. 100, No. 110, No. 120, No. 130, No. 140
Endo-Post	1.1°	Prefabricated Precious Metal Dowel	Smooth	No. 70, No. 80, No. 90, No. 100, No. 110, No. 120, No. 130, No. 140

Diameter scale (in mm.): 0.5 0.6 0.7 0.8 0.9 1.0 1.1 1.2 1.3 1.4 1.5 1.6 1.7 1.8 1.9 2.0 2.1 2.2 2.3 2.4

DIAMETER (in mm.)

DOWEL	TAPER	TYPE	SURFACE	Markings (with approximate diameter in mm)
Gates-Glidden Drill	0°			No. 1 (0.5); No. 2 (0.7); No. 3 (0.9); No. 4 (1.1); No. 5 (1.3); No. 6 (1.5)
Kurer	0°	Pretapped Threaded Steel Dowel	Threaded	No. 00 Reamer / No. 0 Reamer (1.3); No. 00 Shank (1.4); No. 1 Reamer (1.4); No. 0 Shank (1.6); No. 2 Reamer (1.6); No. 1 Shank (1.7); No. 2 Shank (1.8); No. 3 Reamer (1.8); No. 3 Shank (2.0)
NuBond Fast Post	1.6°	Stainless Steel Dowel	Serrated	No. 1 Reamer & Post (0.9); No. 2 Reamer & Post (1.2); No. 3 Reamer & Post (1.4); No. 4 Reamer & Post (1.6); No. 5 Reamer & Post (1.9); No. 6 Reamer & Post (2.2)
Para-Post	0°	Precision Plastic Pattern / Stainless Steel Dowel	Serrated	.036 in. Brown Post (0.8); .040 in. Yellow Post (1.0); .050 in. Red Post (1.3); .060 in. Black Post (1.5); .070 in. Green Post (1.7)
P-D Crown Posts and Sprues	1.6°	Precision Plastic Dowel / Stainless Steel Dowel	Smooth / Serrated	No. 1 Reamer & Posts (1.0); No. 2 Reamer & Posts (1.3); No. 3 Reamer & Posts (1.5); No. 4 Reamer & Posts (1.8); No. 5 Reamer & Posts (1.9); No. 6 Reamer & Posts (2.1); .050 inch Red Post (2.2)
Peeso Reamer	0°			No. 1 Reamer (0.7); No. 2 Reamer (0.9); No. 3 Reamer (1.1); No. 4 Reamer (1.3); No. 5 Reamer (1.5); No. 6 Reamer (1.7)
Radix	0°	Self-Threading Steel Dowel	Threaded	No. 1 Anchor / No. 1 Drill (1.2); No. 2 Anchor (1.3); No. 2 Reamer (1.4); No. 3 Anchor (1.6); No. 3 Reamer (1.7)

Diameter scale (in mm.): 0.5 0.6 0.7 0.8 0.9 1.0 1.1 1.2 1.3 1.4 1.5 1.6 1.7 1.8 1.9 2.0 2.1 2.2 2.3 2.4

The same material can be used for forming the core. This pattern can be direct, i.e. fabricated on the tooth in the mouth, or it can be indirect, i.e. fabricated on a model made from an impression of the tooth in the mouth.

A prefabricated dowel may be a metal dowel to which a custom core is cast. It can be a dowel which can be cemented into the canal with an amalgam or composite core formed around it. Finally, the dowel may be a standardized precision plastic pattern to which a custom core is added before investing and casting. The prefabricated dowel systems each employs reamers, burs, or drills which are matched to the size of that specific dowel (Fig. 1-20). The comparative sizes of the various dowels and instruments can be seen in Table 1-4.

References

1. Prothero, J. H.: *Prosthetic Dentistry,* Chicago, Medico-Dental Publishers, 1921, pp. 1153–1174.

2. Black, G. V.: A method of grafting artificial crowns on roots of teeth. *Mo Dent J,* 1:233–236, 1869.

3. Baumhammers, A.: Simplified technique for a one-unit cast dowel crown. *Dent Dig,* 68:468–472, Oct. 1962.

4. Demas, N. C.: Direct impression for cast Richmond crown using acetate crown forms. *Dent Dig,* 63:258–259, June 1957.

5. Hampson, E. L. and Clarke, J.: The post-retained crown. *Dent Pract & Dent Rec,* 8:130–135, Jan. 1958.

6. Tamarin, A. H.: A new type of Richmond crown. *JADA,* 69:557–559, Nov. 1964.

7. Eissmann, H. F. and Radke, R. A.: Post-endodontic restoration in Cohen, S. and Burns, R. C.: *Pathways of the Pulp,* St. Louis, C. V. Mosby Co., 1976, pp. 537–575.

8. Dawson, P. E.: Pin-retained amalgam. *Dent Clin N Amer,* 14:63–71, Jan. 1970.

9. Barker, B. C. W.: Restoration on non-vital teeth with crowns. *Aust Dent J,* 8:191–200, June 1963.

10. Bartlett, S. O.: Construction of detached core crowns for pulpless teeth in only two sittings. *JADA,* 77:843–845, Oct. 1968.

11. Dewhirst, R. B., Fisher, D. W. and Shillingburg, H. T.: Dowel-core fabrication. *J South Calif Dent Assoc,* 37:444–449, Oct. 1969.

12. Dooley, B. S.: Preparation and construction of post-retention crowns for anterior teeth. *Aust Dent J,* 12:544–550, Dec. 1967.

13. Gutmann, J. L.: Preparation of endodontically treated teeth to receive a post-core restoration. *J Prosthet Dent,* 38:413–419, Oct. 1977.

14. Ruemping, D. R., Lund, M. R. and Schnell, R. J.: Retention of dowels subjected to tensile and torsional forces. *J Prosthet Dent,* 41:159–162, Feb. 1979.

15. Sall, H. D.: Restorative technics for endodontically treated teeth. *Dent Surv,* 53:45–47, Sept. 1977.

16. Taylor, A. G.: Dowel abutment crown. *Roy Canad Dent Corps Quart,* 4:1–4, Jul. 1963.

17. Hirschfeld, Z. and Stern, N.: Post and core–the biomechanical aspect. *Aust Dent J,* 17:467–468, Dec. 1972.

18. Lau, V. S. M.: The reinforcement of endodontically treated teeth. *Dent Clin N Amer,* 20:313–328, Apr. 1976.

19. Rosen, H.: Operative procedures on multilated endodontically treated teeth. *J Prosthet Dent,* 11:973–986, Sept. 1961.

20. Sapone, J. and Lorencki, S. F.: An endodontic-prosthodontic approach to internal tooth reinforcement. *J Prosthet Dent,* 45:164–174, Feb. 1981.

21. Shillingburg, H. T., Fisher, D. W. and Dewhirst, R. B.: Restoration of endodontically treated posterior teeth. *J Prosthet Dent,* 24:401–409, Oct. 1970.

22. Baraban, D. J.: A simplified method for making posts and cores. *J Prosthet Dent,* 24:287–297, Sept. 1970.

23. Caputo, A. A. and Standlee, J. P.: Pins and posts–why, when and how. *Dent Clin N Amer,* 20:299–311, Apr. 1976.

24. Rosenstiel, E.: Impression technique for cast core preparations. *Brit Dent J,* 123:599–600, Dec. 1967.

25. Blair, H. A.: The role of endodontics in restorative dentistry. *Dent Clin N Amer,* 15:619–626, July 1971.

26. Charbeneau, G. T.: Planning for the restoration of non-vital teeth. *J Mich St Dent Assoc,* 42:75–78, Feb. 1960.

27. Frank, A. L.: Protective coronal coverage of the pulpless tooth. *JADA,* 59:895–900, Nov. 1959.

28. Healey, H. J.: Coronal restoration of the treated pulpless tooth. *Dent Clin N Amer,* 1:885–896, Nov. 1957.

29. Segat, L.: Restoration of non-vital teeth. *J Mich St Dent Assoc,* 44:254-259, Sept. 1962.

30. Tidmarsh, B. G.: Restoration of endodontically treated posterior teeth. *J Endo,* 2:374–375, Dec. 1976.

31. Baraban, D. J.: Immediate restoration of pulpless teeth. *J Prosthet Dent,* 28:607–612, Dec. 1972.

32. Baum, L.: Dowel placements in the endodontically treated tooth. *J Conn St Dent Assoc,* 53:116–117, Summer 1979.

33. Henry, P. J. and Bower, R. C.: Post core systems in crown and bridgework. *Aust Dent J,* 22:46–52, Feb. 1977.

34. Johnson, J. K., Schwartz, N. L. and Blackwell, R. T.: Evaluation and restoration of endodontically treated posterior teeth. *JADA,* 93:597–605, Sept. 1976.

35. Perel, M. L. and Muroff, F. I.: Clinical criteria for posts and cores. *J Prosthet Dent,* 28:405–411, Oct. 1972.

36. Waliszewski, K. J. and Sabala, C. L.: Combined endodontic and restorative treatment considerations. *J Prosthet Dent,* 40:152–156, Aug. 1978.

37. Guzy, G. E. and Nicholls, J. I.: In vitro comparison of intact endodontically treated teeth with and without endo-post reinforcement. *J Prosthet Dent,* 42:39–44, Jul. 1979.

38. Kantor, M. E. and Pines, M. S.: A comparative study of restorative techniques for pulpless teeth. *J Prosthet Dent,* 38:405–412, Oct. 1977.

39. Trabert, K. C., Caputo, A. A. and Abou-Rass, M.: Tooth fracture–a comparison of endodontic and restorative treatments. *J Endo,* 4:341–345, Nov. 1978.

40. Colley, I. T., Hampson, E. L. and Lehman, M. L.: Retention of post crowns: An assessment of the relative efficiency of posts of difficult shapes and sizes. *Brit Dent J,* 124:63–69, Jan. 1968.

41. Krupp, J. D., Caputo, A. A., Trabert, K. C. and Standlee, J. P.: Dowel retention with glass ionomer cement. *J Prosthet Dent,* 41:163–166, Feb. 1979.

42. Johnson, J. K. and Sakumura, J. S.: Dowel form and tensile force. *J Prosthet Dent,* 40:645–649, Dec. 1978.

43. Standlee, J. P., Caputo, A. A. and Hanson, E. C.: Retention of endodontic dowels: Effects of cement, dowel length, diameter, and design. *J Prosthet Dent,* 39:401–405, Apr. 1978.

44. Abdullah, S. I., Mohammed, H. and Thayer, K. E.: Restoration of endodontically treated teeth: A review. *J Canad Dent Assoc,* 40:300–303, Apr. 1974.

45. Fellman, S.: Indirect technique for gold core and crown restorations for non-vital teeth. *Dent Surv,* 40:41–43, Mar. 1964.

46. Gentile, D.: Direct dowels for endodontically treated teeth. *Dent Dig,* 71:500–501, Nov. 1965.

47. Greenwald, A. S.: Cast gold post and crown restoration. *Dent Surv,* 41:47–50, Apr. 1965.

48. Healey, H. J.: Restoration of the effectively treated pulpless tooth. *J Prosthet Dent,* 4:842–849, Nov. 1954.

49. Kahn, H., Fishman, I. and Malone, W. F.: A simplified method for constructing a core following endodontic treatment. *J Prosthet Dent,* 37:32–36, Jan. 1977.

50. McPherson, J. L.: Combined endodontic and dowel-type restorative procedures. *Dent Dig,* 77:16–22, Jan. 1971.

51. Miller, A. W.: Direct pattern technique for posts and cores. *J Prosthet Dent,* 40:392–397, Oct. 1978.

52. Mitchell, P. S. and Blass, M. S.: A technique for restoring the pulpless tooth. *J Ga Dent Assoc,* 46:14–17, Summer 1972.

53. Mondelli, J., Piccino, A. C. and Berbert, A.: An acrylic resin pattern for a cast dowel and core. *J Prosthet Dent,* 25:413–417, Apr. 1971.

54. Rosenberg, P. A. and Antonoff, S. J.: Gold posts. Common problems in preparation and technique for fabrication. *NY St Dent J,* 37:601–606, Dec. 1971.

55. Samani, S. I. A. and Harris, W. T.: A procedure for repairing fractured post-core restorations. *J Prosthet Dent,* 39:627–631, Jun. 1978.

56. Silverstein, W. H.: The reinforcement of weakened pulpless teeth. *J Prosthet Dent,* 14:372–381, Mar. 1964.

57. Stahl, G. J. and O'Neal, R. B.: The composite resin dowel and core. *J Prosthet Dent,* 33:642–48, Jun. 1975.

58. Ward, N. L.: Current ideas on post-crown treatment. *Int Dent J,* 12:374–381, Sept. 1962.

59. Welsh, S. L. and Priddy, W. L.: Direct fabrication of interlocking endodontic posts. *J Prosthet Dent,* 39:115–117, Jan. 1978.

60. Wiland, L.: A dimension controlled and accurate procedure for a gold post restoration of an anterior tooth. *Dent Dig,* 72:394–397, Sept. 1966.

61. Yuodelis, R. and Morrison, K.: Full coverage restoration of pulpless anterior and bicuspid teeth. *J Canad Dent Assoc,* 32:516–521, Sept. 1966.

62. Baker, C. R.: The dowel crown. *JADA,* 61:479–83, Oct. 1960.

63. Christy, J. M. and Pipko, D. J.: Fabrication of a dual-post veneer crown. *JADA,* 75:1419–1425, Dec. 1967.

64. Federick, D. R.: A one appointment dowel and core technic. *Dent Surv,* 52:50–51, Dec. 1976.

65. Goerig, A. C. and Mueninghoff, L. A.: Management of the endodontically treated tooth. Part I. Philosophy for restoration design. *J Prosthet Dent,* in press.

66. Hamilton, A. I.: Porcelain dowel crowns. *J Prosthet Dent,* 9:639–644, Jul. 1959.

67. Larato, D. C.: Single unit cast post crown for pulpless anterior tooth roots. *J Prosthet Dent,* 16:145–149, Jan.-Feb. 1966.

68. Lovdahl, P. E. and Dumont, T. D.: A dowel-core technique for multi-rooted teeth. *J Prosthet Dent,* 27:44–47, Jan. 1972.

69. Pickard, H. M.: Variants of the post crown. *Brit Dent J,* 117:517–526, Dec. 1964.

70. Pokorny, M.: Proper dowel preparation for endodontic treatment. *Dent Surv,* 49:36–37, Aug. 1973.

71. Spangler, C. C.: Posts and cores: Some new ideas. *Dent Surv,* 56:33–35, Jun. 1980.

72. Asawa, G. N.: Cast dowel-core fabrication on a pre-existing crown. *Dent Surv,* 48:36–37, Jan. 1972.

73. Jacoby, W. E.: Practical technique for the fabrication of a direct pattern for a post-core restoration. *J Prosthet Dent,* 35:357–360, Mar. 1976.

74. Priest, G. and Goerig, A. C.: Post and core fabrication beneath an existing crown. *J Prosthet Dent,* 42:645–648, Dec. 1979.

75. Burnell, S. C.: Improved cast dowel and base for restoring endodontically treated teeth. *JADA,* 68:39–45, Jan. 1964.

76. Weine, F. S., Kahn, H., Wax, A. H. and Taylor, G. N.: The use of standardized tapered plastic pins in post and core fabrication. *J Prosthet Dent,* 29:542–548, May 1973.

77. Greenberg, M.: Concurrent root canal filling and gold post insertion. *Dent Surv,* 40:39–42, Jul. 1964.

78. Sapone, J.: Endodontic abutment prosthesis. *J Prosthet Dent,* 29:210–216, Feb. 1973.

79. Kayser, A. F.: Prosthodontic aspects of endodontics. *J Prosthet Dent,* 21:645–649, Jun. 1969.

80. Metrick, L.: A direct technique for post-core castings. *J Canad Dent Assoc,* 43:329, Jul. 1977.

81. Shadman, H. and Azarmehr, P.: A direct technique for fabrication of posts and cores. *J Prosthet Dent,* 34:463–466, Oct. 1975.

82. Stern, N. and Hirschfeld, Z.: Principles of preparing endodontically treated teeth for dowel and core restorations. *J Prosthet Dent,* 30:162–165, Aug. 1973.

83. Kurer, P. F.: The Kurer anchor system for post crown restorations. *J Ont Dent Assoc,* 45:57–60, Feb. 1968.

84. Shillingburg, H. T., Kessler, J. C. and Wilson, E. L.: Root dimensions and dowel size. *Calif Dent J,* In press.

85. Henry, P. J.: Photoelastic analysis of post core restorations. *Aust Dent J,* 22:157–159, Jun. 1977.

86. Mazzuchelli, L.: Post and core construction. *Rhode Island Dent J,* 5:11–15, Jun. 1972.

87. Skurnik, H.: Rehabilitation rationale for pulpless teeth. *J Prosthet Dent,* 15:528–542, May-Jun. 1965.

88. Charlton, G.: A prefabricated post and core for porcelain jacket crowns. *Brit Dent J,* 119:452–456, Nov. 1965.

89. Standlee, J. P., Caputo, A. A., Collard, E. W. and Pollack, M. H.: Analysis of stress distribution of endodontic posts. *Oral Surg,* 33:952–960, Jun. 1972.

90. Hanson, E. C. and Caputo, A. A.: Cementing mediums and retentive characteristics. *J Prosthet Dent,* 32:551–557, Nov. 1974.

91. Tilk, M. A., Lommel, T. J. and Gerstein, H.: A study of mandibular and maxillary root widths to determine dowel size. *J Endo,* 5:79–82, Mar. 1979.

92. Durney, E. C. and Rosen, H.: Root fracture as a complication of post design and insertion: A laboratory study. *Oper Dent,* 2:90–96, 1977.

93. Schnell, F. J.: Effect of immediate dowel space preparation on the apical seal of endodontically filled teeth. *Oral Surg,* 45:470–474, Mar. 1978.

94. Neagley, R. L.: The effect of dowel preparation on the apical seal of endodontically treated teeth. *Oral Surg,* 28:739–745, Nov. 1969.

95. Greene, G. S.: Planning the gold post in endodontic treatment. *NY St Dent J,* 30:334–336, Oct. 1964.

96. Hodosh, M. and Mirman, M.: Instrument to aid in placing a "short" silver point prior to post construction. *Dent Dig,* 73:547–549, Dec. 1967.

97. Shaykin, J. B.: Endodontic silver points in tooth reconstruction. *JADA,* 61:363–364, Sept. 1960.

98. Zak, E. L.: Technic to prepare root canals just once for dowel crowns. *Dent Surv,* 50:53–54, Apr. 1974.

99. Goerig, A. C. and Mueninghoff, L. A.: Management of the endodontically treated tooth. Part II. Technique. *J Prosthet Dent,* In press.

100. Colman, H. L.: Restoration of endodontically treated teeth. *Dent Clin N Amer,* 23:647–662, Oct. 1979.

101. Fisher, D. W., Jeannet, D. J., and Kwan, S. K.: An evaluation of methods for preparing teeth to receive retentive posts. *J Dent Res,* Abs no. 532, 61:237, Mar. 1982.

102. McPherson, J. L.: A simplified root-dowel technique. *J South Calif Dent Assoc,* 39:115–119, Feb. 1971.

103. Sheets, C. E.: Dowel and core foundations. *J Prosthet Dent,* 23:58–65, Jan. 1970.

Additional Reading

Arvidson, K. and Johansson, G.: Surface analysis of screwposts. *Scand J Dent Res,* 87:155–158, Apr. 1979.

Barak, M. A.: Immediate post crown for fractured anterior teeth. *Dent Surv,* 34:178–180, Feb. 1958.

Barouch, E.: Preparation and direct wax-up for a gold post on an endodontically treated tooth. *Dent Surv,* 56:48–50, Feb. 1980.

Bower, R. C. and Henry, P. J.: Periodontal considerations in the restoration of non-vital teeth. *Aust Dent J,* 21:527–531, Dec. 1976.

Davy, D. T., Dilley, G. L. and Krejci, R. F.: Determination of stress patterns in root-filled teeth incorporating various dowel designs. *J Dent Res,* in press.

Day, R. C.: Two-part coping, dowel and core. *J Prosthet Dent,* 43:527–529, May 1980.

Derand, T.: The principle stress distribution in a root with a loaded post in model experiments. *J Dent Res,* 56:1463–1467, Dec. 1977.

Ehrmann, E. H. and Feiglin, B.: The obturation of the entire root canal with a dowel crown. *J Endo,* 6:696–701, Aug. 1980.

Hoag, E. P. and Dwyer, T. G.: A comparative evaluation of three post and core techniques. *J Prosthet Dent,* 44:177–181, Feb. 1982.

Kwan, E. H. and Harrington, G. W.: The effect of immediate post preparation on apical seal. *J Endo,* 7:325–329, July 1981.

Leggett, L. J.: Restoration of non-vital posterior teeth. *J Brit Endo Soc,* 12:73–82, Jul. 1979.

Meyer, H. I.: Acrylic dowel crown. *Dent Items Int,* 72:915, 1950.

Myers, A. Q., Kneller, F. and Borden, B. G.: A precise method of preparing posts and coresan evaluation of the BTM Depth Gauge. *Dent Surv,* 56:38–39, Jan. 1980.

Neaverth, E. J. and Kahn, H.: Re-treatment of dowel-obturated root canals. *JADA,* 76:325–328, Feb. 1968.

Petersen, K. B.: Longitudinal root fracture due to corrosion of an endodontic post. *J Canad Dent Assoc,* 37:66–68, Jun. 1971.

Ribbons, J. W.: Use of a composite filling material in periodontal splinting and the construction of cast crowns. *Dent Pract Dent Res,* 22:316–318, Apr. 1972.

Samani, S. I. A. and Harris, W. T.: Provisional restorations for anterior teeth requiring endodontic therapy. *J Endo,* 5:340–343, Nov. 1979.

Scully, B. R.: The tapered dowel pin as a post and core. *J Prosthet Dent,* 27:289–291. Mar. 1972.

Sicklemore, F. A.: Post crowns–some weaknesses. *Brit Dent J,* 107:306, 1959.

Silness, J.: Distribution of corrosion products in teeth restored with metal crowns retained by stainless steel posts. *Acta Odontol Scand,* 37(6):317–321, 1979.

Sotera, A. J.: Creating dentin in nonvital teeth. *Quint Int,* 9:21–27, Aug. 1978.

Waliszewski, K. J.: Restorative techniques available to rehabilitate endodontically treated teeth. *Quint Int,* 10:13–17, Nov. 1979.

Warren, S. R. and Gutmann, J. L.: Simplified method for removing intraradicular posts. *J Prosthet Dent,* 42:353–356, Sep. 1979.

Zmener, O.: Effect of dowel preparation on the apical seal of endodontically treated teeth. *J Endo,* 6:687–690, Aug. 1980.

Chapter 2

Custom Dowel-Core (Direct)

The direct custom dowel-core is made by fabricating a resin or wax pattern in the prepared tooth in the patient's mouth. Some form of plastic dowel or thin metal post is used as the central reinforcement around which the resin or wax pattern is formed. This method of rebuilding endodontically treated teeth has been used for a number of years. Many of the prefabricated precision plastic pattern systems make use of the concept of the dowel-core. They differ from the custom dowel-core principally by eliminating the relining of the dowel in the canal.

Relining the dowel, while it does take time, provides for an accurate fit of the dowel in the canal, with faciolingual irregularities in the canal incorporated into the anti-rotational aspect of the dowel. When the canal is not ovoid enough to provide the needed anti-rotational stability, the canal preparation is modified with keyways to resist torque in the restoration.

The pattern can be made of wax, reinforced with a plastic rod,[1-3] a bur,[4,5] a metal pin,[6,7] or a paper clip.[8] An acrylic resin* can also be used for this purpose,[9-20] or wax and acrylic can be combined.[21,22] The use of resin allows the pattern to be formed into a well adapted, solid dowel that can be manipulated easily in the mouth without becoming distorted or loose in the canal.

At one time, dowel-cores were usually made of a hard gold alloy, but the recent increase in the cost of gold makes this impractical for most cases. Base metal alloys have been used for this purpose.[11,23,24] Although nickel-chrome alloys were originally chosen for economic reasons, their hardness and high yield strength make them an excellent choice for the job.

Peeso reamers** are used for the enlargement of the canal[1,3,8,9,16,21,22] because of their non-cutting tip and their

---

* Duralay, Reliance Dental Mfg. Co., Chicago, IL.

** Peeso reamers, Union Broach Corporation, Long Island City, NY.

ability to stay within the confines of the canal. The size of the largest reamer to be used on a tooth (and therefore the diameter of the dowel) will be deter- mined by the size of the tooth. Average reamer size is presented in Table 2-1 (see pages 30 and 31 for tooth and dowel sizes).

TABLE 2-1 **Peeso Reamer Sizes**

Reamer Number	Diameter	Teeth
1	0.7 mm.	Mandibular incisor
2	0.9 mm.	Maxillary first premolar Maxillary second molar (DF) Mandibular first molar (ML) Mandibular second molar (MF, ML)
3	1.1 mm.	Maxillary second premolar Maxillary first molar (MF, DF) Maxillary second molar (MF) Mandibular first molar (MF, D) Mandibular second molar (D)
4	1.3 mm.	Maxillary lateral incisor Mandibular premolar Maxillary molar (L)
5	1.5 mm.	Canine
6	1.7 mm.	Maxillary central incisor

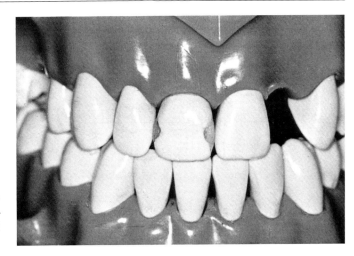

Fig. 2-1 The need for a dowel-core is predicated in part on damage to the crown from caries and previous restorations.

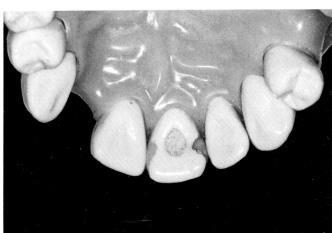

Fig. 2-2 Destruction of tooth structure is inescapably increased by the endodontic access on the lingual surface.

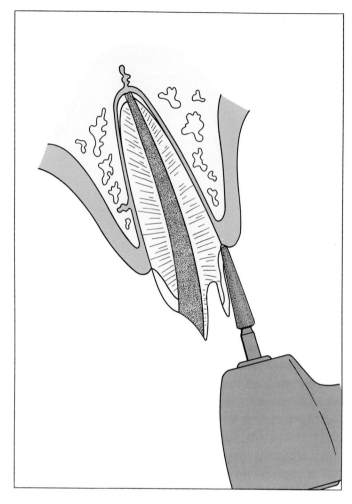

Fig. 2-3 The preparation for the final restoration, which is usually a porcelain fused to metal crown for an anterior tooth, will be roughly approximated first.

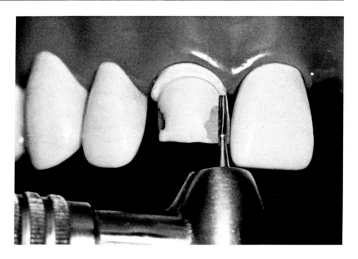

Fig. 2-4 Following incisal reduction of 2.0 mm., the facial axial surfaces are reduced to a depth of 1.25 mm. with a flat-end tapered diamond. The surface is smoothed with a No. 170 nondentate tapered fissure bur, emphasizing the gingival shoulder at the same time. Bases, old restorations, and caries are ignored at this time.

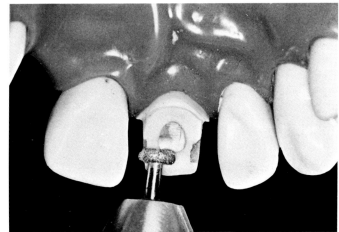

Fig. 2-5 The first step in the reduction of the lingual surface is accomplished by hollow grinding the cingulum to a depth of 1.0 mm. This will produce a distinctly concave surface.

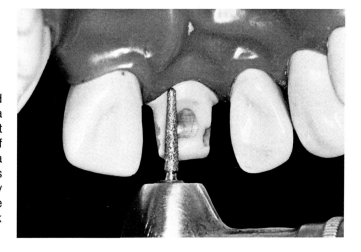

Fig. 2-6 A round-end tapered diamond is used to produce a chamfer finish line on the upright segment of the lingual surface. If the cingulum wall is too short, a shoulder will be prepared. This will lengthen the lingual wall by moving it facially toward the center of the tooth where the bulk of tooth structure is greater.

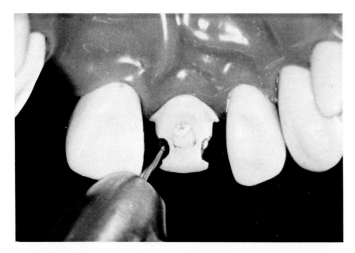

Fig. 2-7 Once the porcelain fused to metal preparation has been roughed out, the previous restorations, bases, and any remaining caries are removed with a No. 4 or No. 6 round bur.

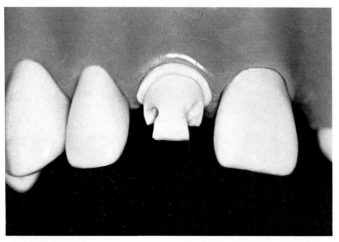

Fig. 2-8 Evaluate the remaining tooth structure to determine how much must be removed. Remaining coronal tooth structure increases the dowel length and adds to the strength of the crown by allowing a wide band or "ferrule" to be formed by the final crown.[25]

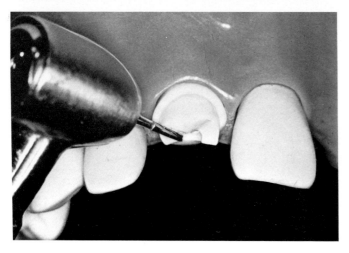

Fig. 2-9 Remove any thin, unsupported or questionable tooth structure with a No. 170 nondentate tapered fissure bur. Also remove any undercut areas that may remain in the coronal portion of the canal preparation. It is unnecessary and undesirable to remove all supragingival coronal tooth structure.

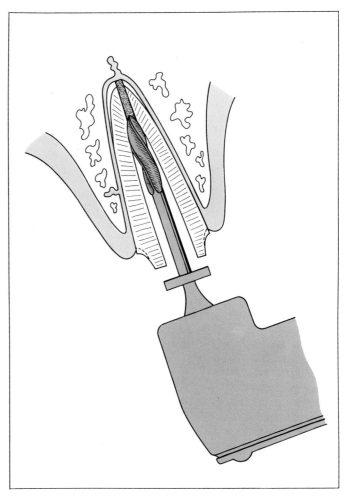

Fig. 2-10 The tooth is now ready for preparation of the dowel space. The instrument of choice for enlarging the canal is a Peeso reamer. Its sharp, non-cutting tip will follow the path of least resistance, the gutta percha in the canal.

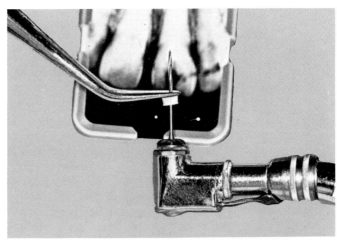

Fig. 2-11 A Peeso reamer is measured against a radiogaph of the tooth being restored to determine the length to which the reamer will be inserted into the canal. Slide a rubber stop onto the reamer to serve as an indicator of preparation depth.

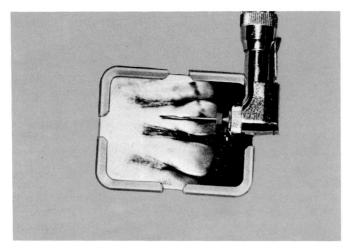

Fig. 2-12 Move the stop to the place on the reamer that will correspond with the landmark when the reamer is inserted to the proper depth in the canal. The dowel should be two-thirds the length of the canal, and at least as long as the crown. Do not come any closer than 4.0 mm. from the apex.

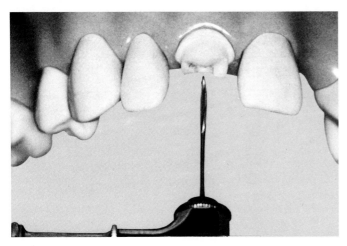

Fig. 2-13 After removing as much gutta percha as possible with a hot endodontic plugger, begin the actual canal preparation with the largest reamer which will fit into the canal. Make a radiograph to check the accuracy of the preparation depth. Use the radiograph to make any necessary adjustments in the reamer length.

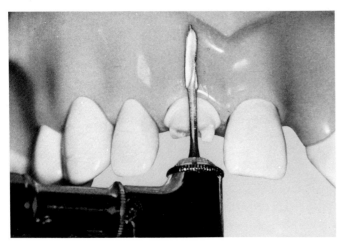

Fig. 2-14 Continue enlarging the canal with graduated sizes of reamers until the size is reached which has been selected for the tooth being restored. A No. 6 reamer is shown superimposed over the tooth.

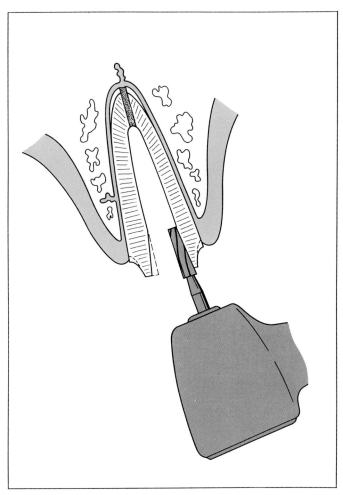

Fig. 2-15   A keyway is placed in the orifice of the canal to provide anti-rotational stability to the dowel.[1, 3, 5, 20, 21, 22, 26] One or more vertical grooves are cut in the walls of the canals, extending 3–4 mm. down the canal. The same effect can be achieved on a multi-rooted tooth by placing a short dowel into a second canal.[27]

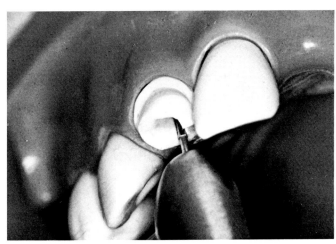

Fig. 2-16   The keyway should be cut to the depth of the diameter of a No. 170 bur (approximately 1.0 mm.) in the area of greatest bulk. A second opposing keyway is placed in larger teeth.

53

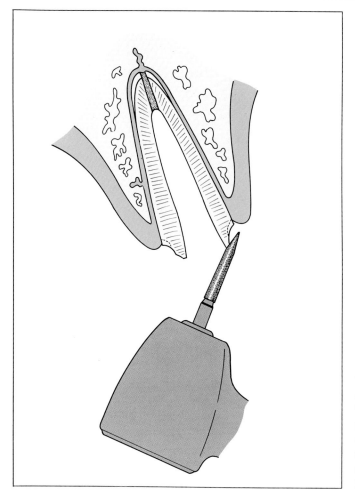

Fig. 2-17   Add a prominent contrabevel to provide a collar around the occlusal circumference of the preparation. It will aid in holding the tooth together and preventing fracture. This serves as a safeguard on a precision fitting dowel, which can exert lateral forces during cementation.

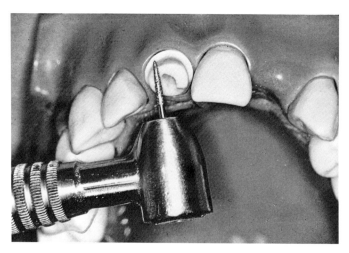

Fig. 2-18   A wide, distinct bevel is placed around the occlusal external periphery of the preparation with a flame diamond.

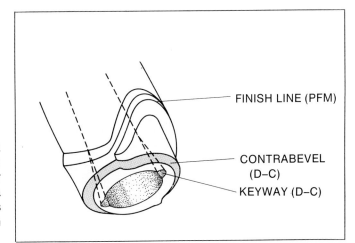

Fig. 2-19 The features of a dowel-core preparation on an anterior tooth. The finish line for the final restoration, in this case a porcelain fused to metal crown, is always placed on solid tooth structure.

FINISH LINE (PFM)

CONTRABEVEL (D–C)

KEYWAY (D–C)

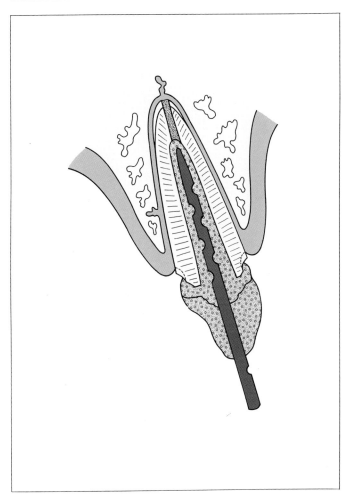

Fig. 2-20 The dowel-core pattern will be fabricated with a plastic sprue and resin.

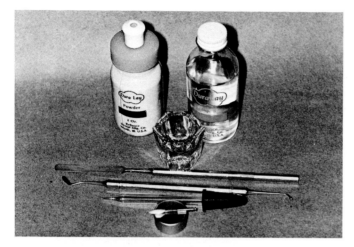

Fig. 2-21 Armamentarium for the dowel-core pattern: Duralay monomer and polymer,* a dappen dish, spatula, plastic instrument, medicine dropper, lubricant (petrolatum), and Peeso reamer with cotton pellet.

* Duralay, Reliance Dental Mfg. Co., Chicago, IL.

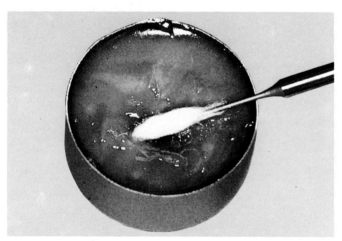

Fig. 2-22 Wrap a cotton pellet tightly around a No. 1 Peeso reamer and dip it into the Duralay lubricant. The cotton should be completely coated with lubricant.

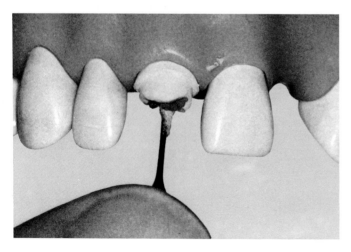

2-23 Insert the Peeso reamer with lubricant covered cotton pellet into the canal. Make sure that it extends the full length of the dowel preparation. Wait a few seconds for it to warm to body temperature. Then pump the reamer in and out to make sure that the entire canal is *well* coated. Some of the lubricant should be on the coronal part of the preparation as well.

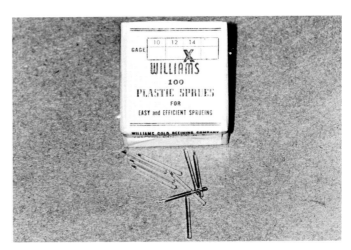

Fig. 2-24 Use 14 gauge plastic sprues* for the pattern. They are hard enough to reinforce the pattern, and they will burn out cleanly. Plastic toothpicks are softened by the monomer and often are separated from the pattern during removal.

* Williams Gold Refining Co., Inc., Buffalo, NY.

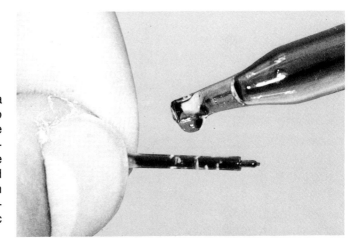

Fig. 2-25 Trim the sprue with a garnet disc so that it will fit into the canal easily. It must reach the apical end of the dowel preparation. Cut a small notch in the facial portion of the occlusal end of the plastic sprue to aid in orienting the pattern in subsequent steps. Coat the plastic sprue with monomer.

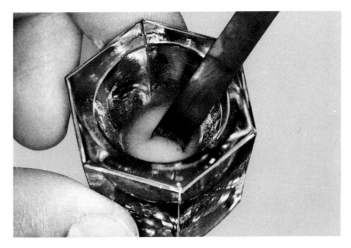

Fig. 2-26 Mix the Duralay monomer and polymer to a thin, runny consistency in a dappen dish.

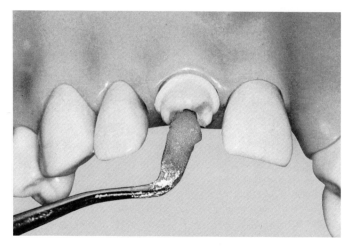

Fig. 2-27 Fill the mouth of the lubricated canal as completely as possible with Duralay applied with an IPPA plastic filling instrument.

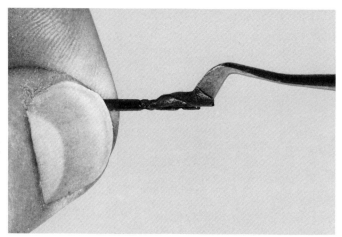

Fig. 2-28 Coat the plastic sprue with the acrylic while it is still fluid.

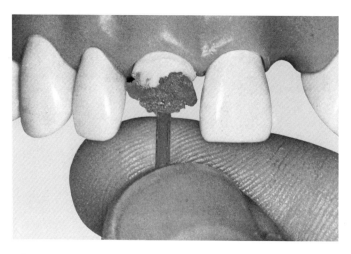

Fig. 2-29 Seat the resin covered sprue in the canal until it has touched the apical end of the dowel preparation. Make sure that all of the external contrabevel is covered at this time. It will be difficult to do later without interfering with the fit of the dowel pattern in the canal.

Fig. 2-30 More resin is added to the coronal portion of the pattern to provide the bulk for the core. It can be added while the dowel is still polymerizing, or it can be added as a fresh mix to the polymerized dowel. When the resin on the dowel itself becomes doughy, pump the pattern up and down to prevent its being locked into any undercuts in the canal. Remove the dowel from the canal and see if it extends the full length of the prepared canal. Fill any voids with soft utility wax and replace the pattern.

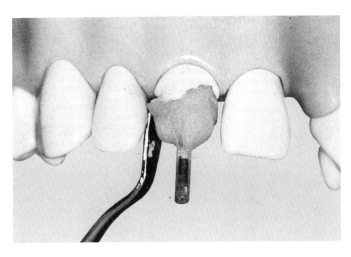

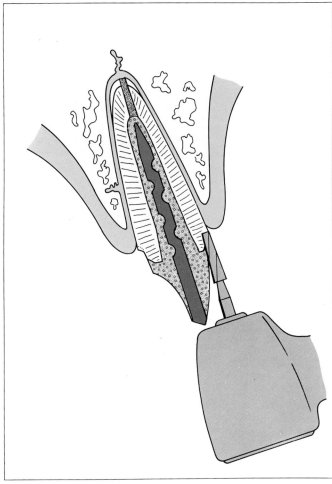

Fig. 2-31 Shape the coronal portion of the pattern to form it into a crown preparation for the final restoration.

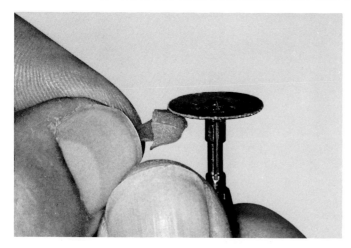

Fig. 2-32 Remove the pattern from the mouth and roughly shape the axial surfaces with a garnet disc. Replace it in the tooth from time to time to insure that the contours being shaped are consistent with the remaining coronal tooth structure. Be sure that the finish line of the final crown preparation is on tooth structure and not on the core.

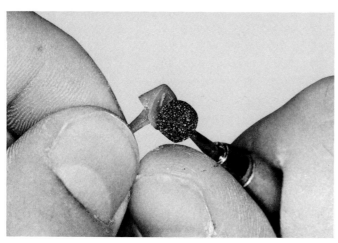

Fig. 2-33 Grind the concave lingual surface incisal to the cingulum with a large, barrel-shaped green stone. Replace it in the mouth to check for clearance with the opposing teeth. The finishing touches can be applied to the pattern with a nondentate tapered fissure bur, after the pattern has been seated on the tooth. It is very important to complete the reduction and contouring in acrylic because it is very difficult and time-consuming to shape the nickel-chrome dowel-core after it has been cast.

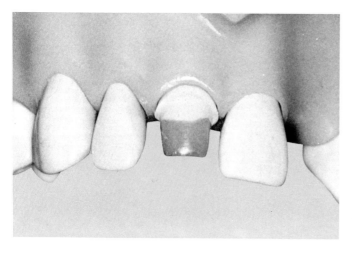

Fig. 2-34 Labial view of the completed Duralay pattern in place in the tooth.

Fig. 2-35 The lingual surface of the pattern exhibits a very short, upright cingulum wall and a concave lingual surface incisal to that. The axial surfaces of the core portion of the pattern should exhibit a smooth, uninterrupted continuation of the contours of the coronal tooth structure.

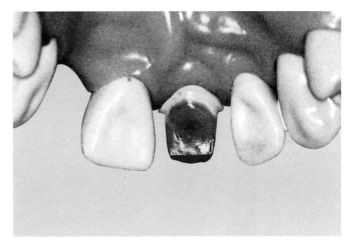

Fig. 2-36 The completed dowel-core pattern has an essentially parallel-sided dowel with a slight taper in the apical area. The apparent taper in the dowel near its junction with the core is caused by the winglike projections of acrylic resin that fill the keyways.

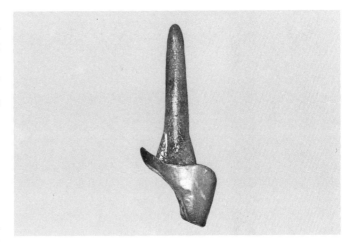

Fig. 2-37 The pattern is attached to a crucible former with a 10 gauge plastic sprue. Sticky wax is used to attach the sprue to the occlusal end of the pattern. If the dowel-core is to be cast in a nickel-chrome alloy, it is invested in a carbon-free phosphate-bonded investment.* Carbon in the mold could produce brittleness in the chromium. If the dowel-core is to be cast in a gold alloy, gypsum investment** is used.

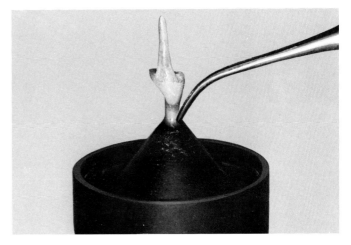

 * High-Temp Investment, Whip-Mix Corporation, Louisville, KY.
** Beauty-Cast Investment, Whip-Mix Corporation, Louisville, KY.

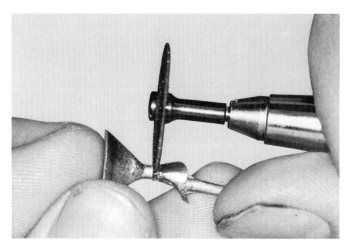

Fig. 2-38 Remove the sprue with a 7/8 inch Carborundum disc or a 1½ inch diameter cut-off disc.

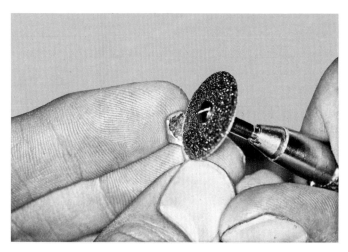

Fig. 2-39 Do the rough trimming with the Carborundum disc and then finish the contouring of the surfaces around the sprue with a No. 8 aluminum oxide pink wheel on a mandrel.

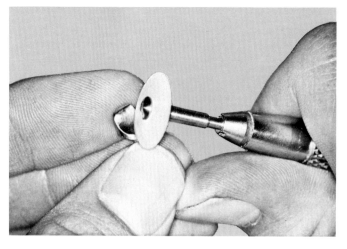

Fig. 2-40 The core portion of the casting should be smoothed to a satin or matte finish with a Burlew* or a white Dedeco "Flexie"** wheel.

* Burlew Wheel, J. F. Jelenko & Co., New Rochelle, NY.
** Dedeco White "Flexie" Wheel, Dental Development & Mfg. Corp., Brooklyn, NY.

Fig. 2-41 Use a No. 34 carbide bur to cut a v-shaped cement escape vent on the side of the dowel. This groove should help greatly to prevent damaging lateral stresses during cementation.[28] In using the hard nickel-chrome alloys, this task can be made easier and faster by placing the groove in the Duralay pattern and retouching it in the finished casting.

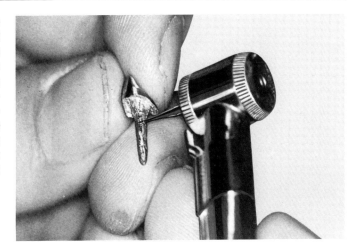

Fig. 2-42 Prepare a thin mix of zinc phosphate cement and insert some into the mouth of the dried, isolated canal. Cover the blade of the instrument with cement a second time and hold it incisal to the mouth of the canal. Insert a slowly rotating Lentulo spiral paste filler through the mass of liquid cement to carry the cement into the canal. In a few seconds, the Lentulo spiral should have coated the walls of the canal. Apply more cement to the mouth of the canal until no more will move into the canal.

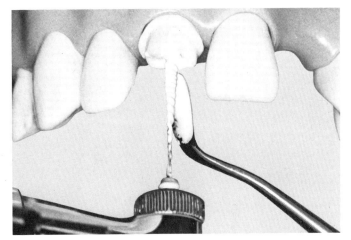

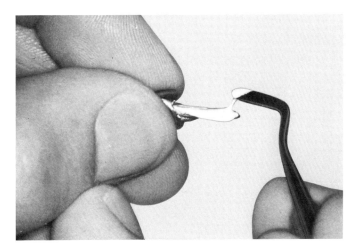

Fig. 2-43 Liberally coat the dowel with the fluid cement and insert the dowel into the canal.

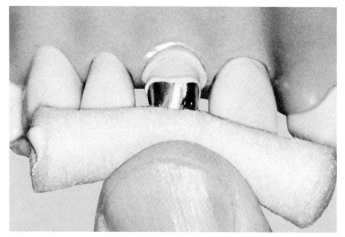

Fig. 2-44 Seat the dowel slowly with finger pressure, allowing the cement to escape ahead of the dowel. If the incisal edge of the core is uncomfortable against the finger, cushion it with a cotton roll. Never mallet a dowel to place. The close fitting hydraulic chamber formed by a custom dowel moving through a viscous liquid in a parallel walled canal can produce considerable stress in the lateral walls of the tooth, and fracture could result.

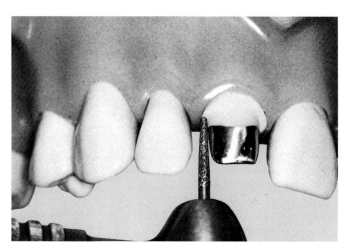

Fig. 2-45 When the cement has set, go over the axial surfaces of the core and tooth structure with a fine grit diamond. It is important to remove any minor undercuts in the axial surfaces near the margin of the dowel-core. If allowed to remain, any defects in the axial surface could present obstacles to the successful completion of the final restoration.

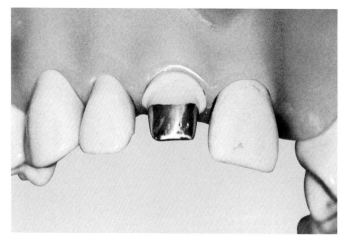

Fig. 2-46 Labial view of the completed dowel-core on a central incisor. Approximately the incisal 60% of the crown preparation is composed of the core.

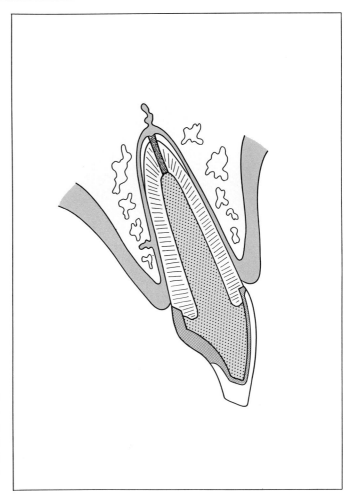

Fig. 2-47 The tooth can now be restored with a crown. That portion of coronal tooth form that has been built up with the core can be treated as though it were tooth structure when the final restoration is fabricated.

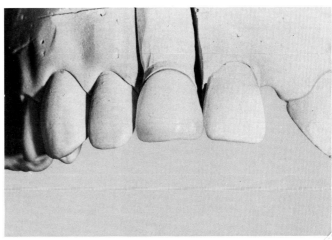

Fig. 2-48 An impression is made of the tooth and a die and working cast are made in the usual way. The coping for the porcelain fused to metal crown is then fabricated on the die, with the porcelain being fused to it.

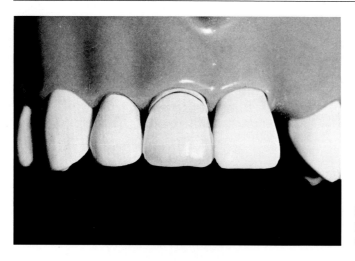

Fig. 2-49 The completed restoration is cemented to the dowel-
core bolstered preparation.

Fig. 2-50 Posterior teeth can also be restored with dowel-cores. Mandibular premolars are treated in the same way as anterior teeth. In maxillary premolars with two canals, a normal length dowel is placed in the longest, straightest, bulkiest root. A short dowel is used as a keyway in the second dowel.

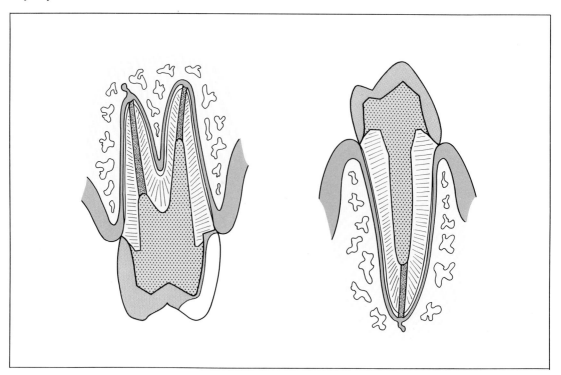

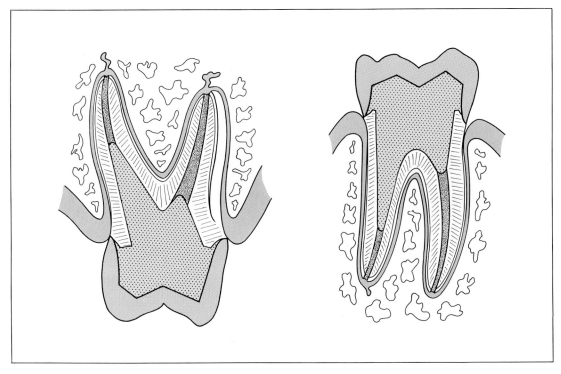

Fig. 2-51 Although single-piece dowel-cores are done frequently on premolars, they are done only rarely on molars. When they are used on molars, the palatal canal is used on maxillary molars and distal canals on mandibular molars.

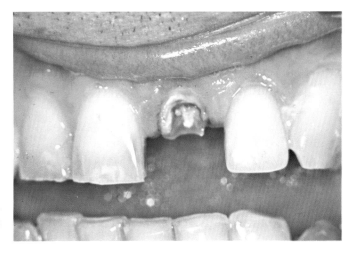

Fig. 2-52 This patient presented with an endodontically treated incisor whose crown and previous core had broken off.

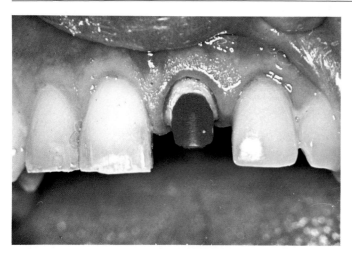

Fig. 2-53 A resin dowel-core pattern is shown in place in the tooth upon completion of fabrication.

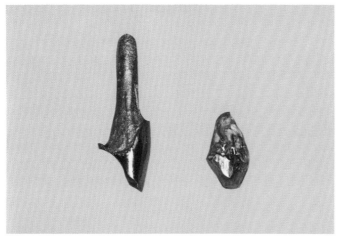

Fig. 2-54 The new dowel-core (left) is compared with the old one (right). The failure of the original dowel-core was undoubtedly due to the extremely short dowel.

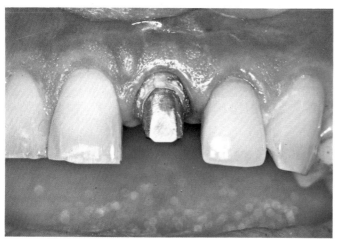

Fig. 2-55 The completed dowel-core is cemented in the tooth. In this particular case, the upright coronal tooth structure so vital for retention of the crown has been completely replaced by the core. This restoration, and others in the series, were restored when gold alloys were being utilized for this purpose.

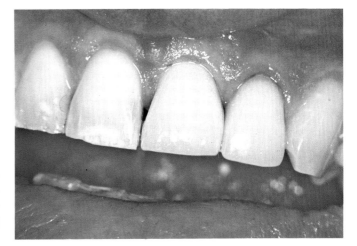

Fig. 2-56 The tooth was restored to function with an acceptable cosmetic result by substituting a dowel-core for the missing coronal tooth structure.

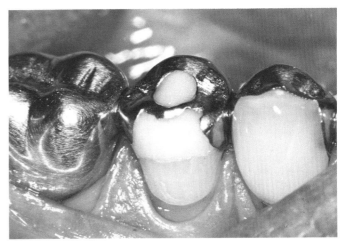

Fig. 2-57 This mandibular premolar was endodontically treated and temporarily restored years after the placement of an M.O.D. onlay.

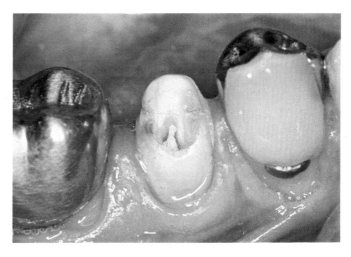

Fig. 2-58 There is virtually no tooth structure remaining on the facial after the onlay, bases, and temporary restorations have been removed. Some substitute for the missing tooth structure must be found. Amalgam pin cores are seldom used for premolars because there is inadequate tooth structure peripheral to the canal in which pins can be safely placed.

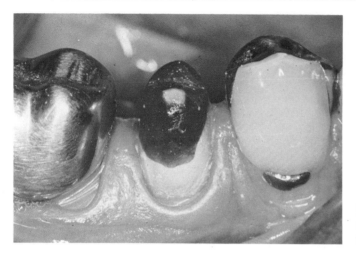

Fig. 2-59 The completed resin dowel-core pattern is seated in the tooth.

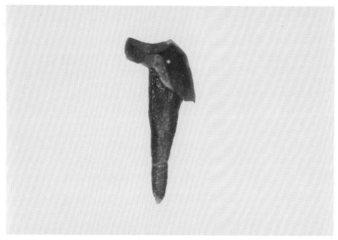

Fig. 2-60 A proximal view of the finished dowel-core pattern shows the utilization of an irregular shape in the occlusal half of the dowel preparation as an anti-rotational device. Almost all of the facial portion of the crown preparation has been replaced by the core, while less than a third of the lingual surface will be part of the core.

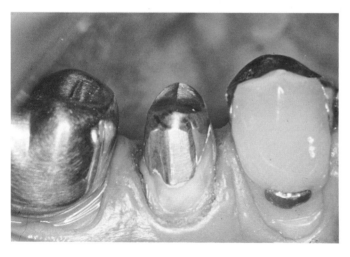

Fig. 2-61 The completed dowel is cemented in the canal. The highly polished surface of the core will be eliminated by the application of finishing stones and pumice.

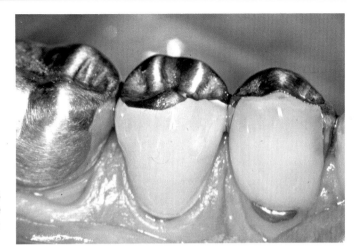

Fig. 2-62 The restored tooth is shown after cementation of the final restoration: a porcelain fused to metal crown.

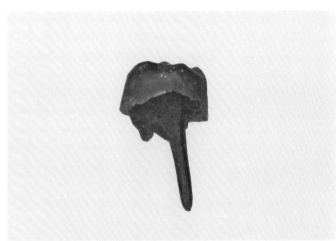

Fig. 2-63 This dowel-core pattern for a mandibular molar shows a long dowel for the distal canal and a short, anti-rotational dowel for the mesial canal.

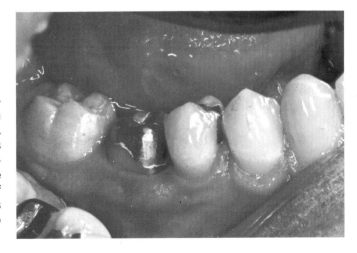

Fig. 2-64 The finished dowel-core is shown after cementation in the mandibular first molar. A dowel-core was selected in this instance because there was virtually no coronal tooth structure remaining. Some build-up of tooth structure with a dowel was needed to provide resistance to horizontally directed forces.

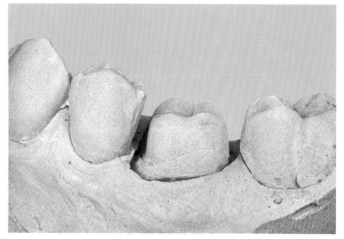

Fig. 2-65 When seen on the working cast, the tooth with the dowel-core looks like an ideal crown preparation in sound tooth structure. The dowel-core margin can be seen on the mesial aspect of the facial surface, slightly occlusal to the gingival finish line of the full crown preparation.

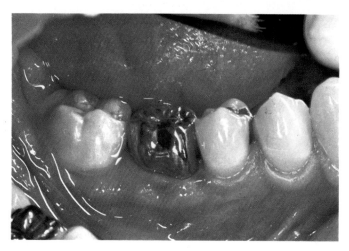

Fig. 2-66 The completed full crown restoration after cementation.

References

1. Barker, B. C. W.: Restoration of non-vital teeth with crowns. *Aust Dent J,* 8:191–200, Jun. 1963.

2. Gentile, D.: Direct dowels for endodontically treated teeth. *Dent Dig,* 71:500–501, Nov. 1965.

3. Silverstein, W. H.: The reinforcement of weakened pulpless teeth. *J Prosthet Dent,* 14:372–381, Mar. 1964.

4. Dill, G. C.: Cast dowel and core techniques. *West Va Dent J,* 44:80–81, Oct. 1970.

5. Rosen, H.: Operative procedures on mutilated endodontically treated teeth. *J Prosthet Dent,* 11:973–986, Sept. 1961.

6. Holt, J. K.: Anterior post crowns. *Brit Dent J,* 113:299–304, Nov. 1962.

7. Metrick, L.: Root canal obliteration with a post crown. *J Canad Dent Assoc,* 27:585–586, Sept. 1961.

8. Taylor, A. G.: Dowel abutment crown. *Roy Canad Dent Corps Quart,* 4:1–4, Jul. 1963.

9. Dewhirst, R. B., Fisher, D. W. and Shillingburg, H. T.: Dowel-core fabrication. *J South Calif Dent Assoc,* 37:444–449, Oct. 1969.

10. Bartlett, S. O.: Construction of detached core crowns for pulpless teeth in only two sittings. *JADA,* 77:843–845, Oct. 1968.

11. DeDomenico, R. J.: Technique for the fabrication of a cast post and core with nonprecious metal. *JADA,* 94:1139–1141, Jun. 1977.

12. Henry, P. J. and Bower, R. C.: Post core systems in crown and bridgework. *Aust Dent J,* 22:46–52, Feb. 1977.

13. Jacoby, W. E.: Practical technique for the fabrication of a direct pattern for a post-core restoration. *J Prosthet Dent,* 35:357–360, Mar. 1976.

14. Mondelli, J., Piccino, A. C. and Berbert, A.: An acrylic resin pattern for a cast dowel and core. *J Prosthet Dent,* 25:413, Apr. 1971.

15. Ram, Z.: T-pins in a direct pattern technique for posts and cores. *J Prosthet Dent,* 40:103–106, Jul. 1978.

16. Rosenberg, P. A. and Antonoff, S. J.: Gold posts. Common problems in preparation and technique for fabrication. *NY St Dent J,* 37:601–606, Dec. 1971.

17. Samani, S. I. A. and Harris, W. T.: A procedure for repairing fractured post-core restorations. *J. Prosthet Dent,* 39:627–631, Jun. 1978.

18. Stern, N.: A direct pattern technique for posts and cores. *J Prosthet Dent,* 28:279–283, Sept. 1972.

19. Waldman, P. M.: Esthetic temporary crowns for devitalized teeth utilizing a resin post. *Dent Dig,* 74:470–471, Nov. 1968.

20. Wiland, L.: A dimension controlled and accurate procedure for a gold post restoration of an anterior tooth. *Dent Dig,* 72:394–397, Sept. 1966.

21. Metrick, L.: A direct technique for post-core castings. *J Canad Dent Assoc,* 43:329, Jul. 1977.

22. Miller, A. W.: Direct pattern technique for posts and cores. *J Prosthet Dent,* 40:392–397, Oct. 1978.

23. Dale, J. W. and Moser, J.: A clinical evaluation of semiprecious alloys for dowels and cores. *J Prosthet Dent,* 38:161–164, Aug. 1977.

24. Pinkley, V. A. and Morris, D. R.: Use of nonprecious metal for cast dowel and core. *J Prosthet Dent,* 32:78–79, Jul. 1974.

25. Eissmann, H. F. and Radke, R. A.: Post-endodontic restoration. In Cohen, S. and Burns, R. C.: *Pathways of the Pulp,* St. Louis, C. V. Mosby Co., 1976, pp. 537–575.

26. Hannah, C. M. D.: Prefabricated post and core patterns. *J Prosthet Dent,* 30:37–42, Jul. 1973.

27. Shillingburg, H. T., Fisher, D. W. and Dewhirst, R. B.: Restoration of endodontically treated posterior teeth, *J Prosthet Dent,* 24:401–409, Oct. 1970.

28. Standlee, J. P., Caputo, A. A., Collard, E. W. and Pollack, M. H.: Analysis of stress distribution of endodontic posts. *Oral Surg,* 33:952–960, Jun. 1972.

Chapter 3

Custom Dowel-Core (Indirect)

A custom dowel-core can also be fabricated by making a wax or resin pattern on a cast of the prepared tooth. This has the advantage of allowing someone besides the dentist to make the pattern, saving chair time in the process. A custom dowel-core can be fabricated in this way, as can the dowel-cores made from many of the prefabricated precision plastic pattern systems.

An impression can be made by injecting impression material into the canal and then using a Lentulo spiral paste filler to insure the elimination of entrapped air and voids in the impression of the canal.[1-3] The impression is reinforced with some type of rigid dowel. Among the items which have been used for this purpose are paper clips,[4, 5] short lengths of wire,[1, 6, 7] plastic sprues,[8] and a root canal instrument (which is also used for placing the impression material).[9] These reinforcing devices not only strengthen the impression when it is made, but also when it is poured and separated.

A custom acrylic dowel can also be made in the tooth, to serve as the impression of the canal in transferring it to a cast for fabrication of the core and restoration.[10] When the indirect technique is used with one of the prefabricated precision plastic patterns, a dowel pattern is placed into the canal, and it is picked up in the impression. The dowel then creates its own space in the cast when the impression is poured.

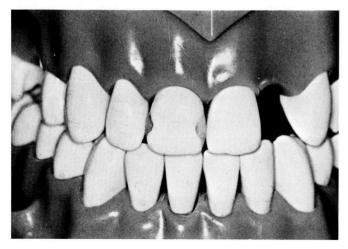

Fig. 3-1 A dowel-core is needed for this tooth because the external destruction required for a crown preparation and the internal destruction required for endodontic treatment leave coronal tooth structure which is compromised both in quantity and in strength.

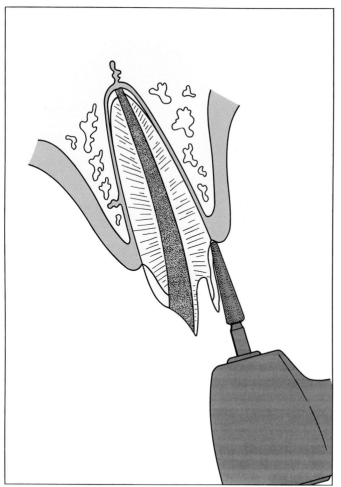

Fig. 3-2 If valuable coronal tooth structure is to be saved, it is necessary to precede the dowel preparation with the crown preparation for the porcelain fused to metal crown.

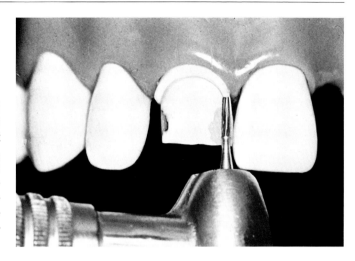

Fig. 3-3 Incisal reduction of 2.0 mm. and facial reduction of 1.25 mm. are accomplished without any regard for old restorations, bases, or caries. Use a flat-end tapered diamond for the bulk reduction, and a No. 170 nondentate tapered fissure bur for finishing and accentuation of the shoulder.

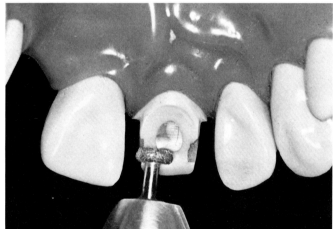

Fig. 3-4 Lingual reduction is begun by cutting the cingulum to a depth of 1.0 mm. with a small wheel diamond. The resultant surface will be distinctly concave.

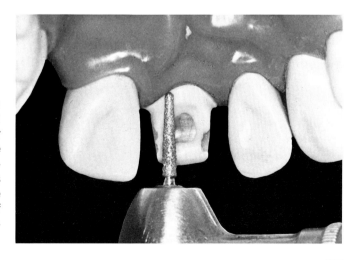

Fig. 3-5 An upright cingulum wall is produced with a round-end tapered diamond. The chamfer finish line that occurs can be changed to a shoulder if the vertical lingual wall is too short. This causes the lingual wall to be moved facially into the center of the tooth, where the wall will become longer.

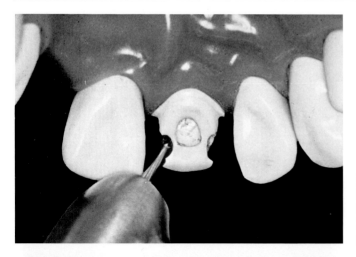

Fig. 3-6 Now that the porcelain fused to metal preparation has been approximated, all caries, bases and old restorations can be removed with a large round bur.

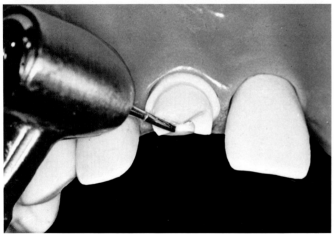

Fig. 3-7 Evaluate the remaining coronal tooth structure and remove the unsupported portion. Leaving coronal tooth structure will make the dowel longer, and the axial contours of the crown preparation will simplify the contouring of the core. Remove thin, unsupported tooth structure with the No. 170 bur.

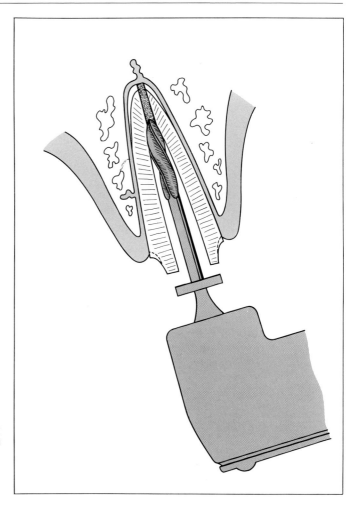

Fig. 3-8 Canal enlargement and preparation will be carried out with a set of Peeso reamers.[3, 4, 8, 11] Their sharp non-cutting tip will follow the canal with minimal risk of lateral perforation.

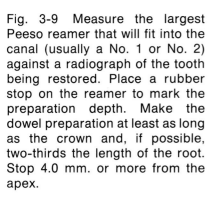

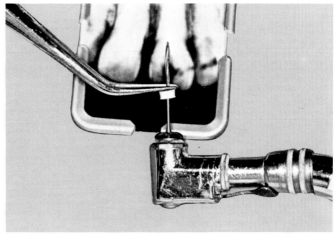

Fig. 3-9 Measure the largest Peeso reamer that will fit into the canal (usually a No. 1 or No. 2) against a radiograph of the tooth being restored. Place a rubber stop on the reamer to mark the preparation depth. Make the dowel preparation at least as long as the crown and, if possible, two-thirds the length of the root. Stop 4.0 mm. or more from the apex.

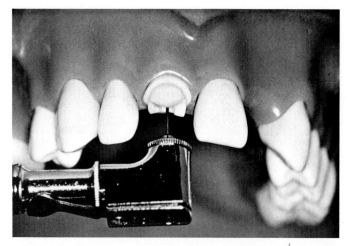

Fig. 3-10   Use a hot endodontic plugger to remove as much gutta percha as possible. Begin the dowel preparation with as large a Peeso reamer as will possibly fit into the canal. If a small tooth or one with a slightly curved root is to be restored, begin the canal enlargement with a Gates Glidden drill. Make a radiograph and use it to make necessary adjustments in reamer length.

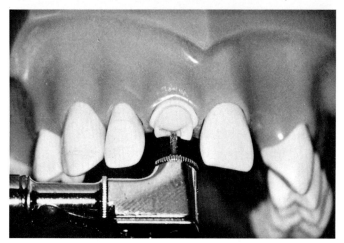

Fig. 3-11   Enlarge the canal with graduated sizes of reamers until the appropriate diameter for the tooth has been reached. To eliminate any possible undercuts, withdraw the Peeso reamer with a slight flaring or leaning motion at the canal orifice.

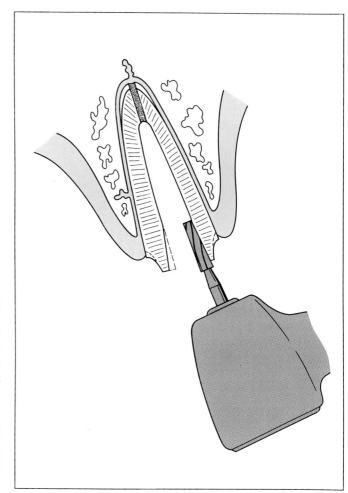

Fig. 3-12 Place a keyway in the mouth of the canal to provide resistance against twisting of the dowel.[3, 7] There is a possibility that its use could endanger the structural integrity of the root.[10] It should not extend too far toward the periphery of the tooth, and there should be no more than one in teeth with small roots. The same effect can be obtained in a multi-rooted tooth by using a short dowel in a second canal.

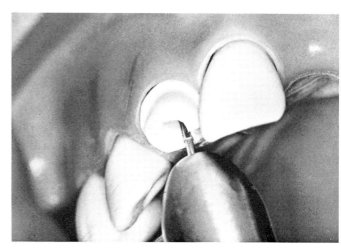

Fig. 3-13 The keyway, a vertical groove, is placed to the length of the cutting blades of the No. 170 bur, and to the depth of the bur's diameter.

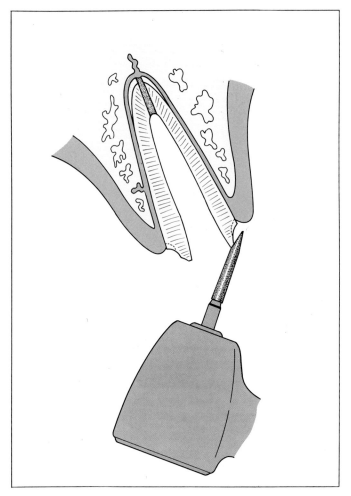

Fig. 3-14   Add a distinct contra-bevel around the occlusal circumference of the dowel-core preparation. This will provide a collar which will help hold the tooth together and prevent fracture.

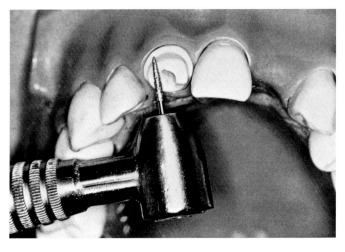

Fig. 3-15   A flame diamond is used to place a wide bevel around the occlusal external periphery of the dowel-core preparation.

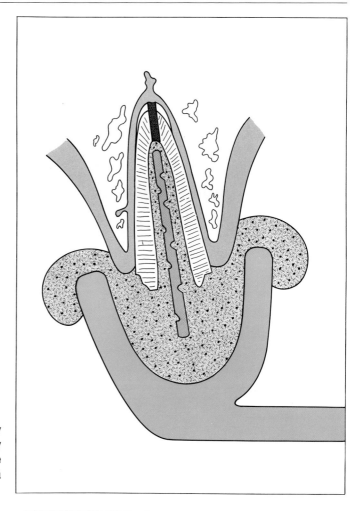

Fig. 3-16 The tooth is now ready for an impression, made with any of the elastomeric materials. The dowel is reinforced with wire or a plastic pin.

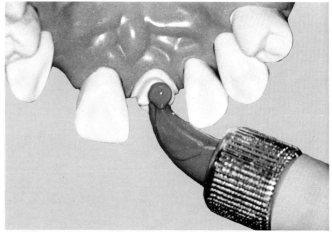

Fig. 3-17 Impression material is injected into the mouth of the canal. While any material with which the operator is familiar can be used, the lighter bodied more flexible materials are probably easier to manipulate. Syringe consistency silicone, either conventional or vinyl polysiloxane, is excellent.

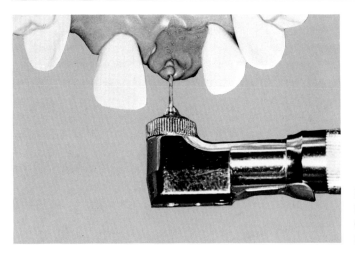

Fig. 3-18 A Lentulo spiral cement filler is inserted into the canal for a few seconds to eliminate as many voids as possible.

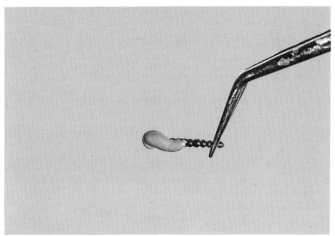

Fig. 3-19 A short length of paper clip, long enough to protrude from the canal, is painted with the adhesive specific for the type of impression material used. Grasping it in cotton pliers, dip it into the impression material on the pad.

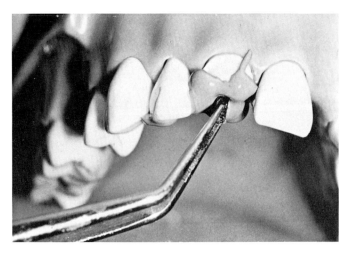

Fig. 3-20 Insert the impression coated wire into the canal, making sure it goes all the way to the apical end of the dowel preparation.

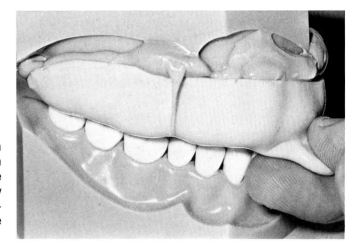

Fig. 3-21 Insert the impression tray and stabilize it in position until the polymerization of the material is complete. Withdraw the impression in the same direction as the path of insertion of the dowel preparation.

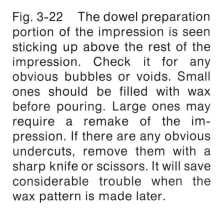
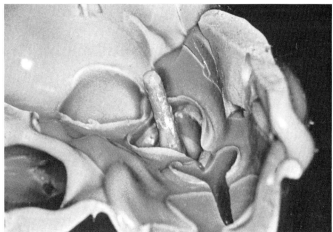

Fig. 3-22 The dowel preparation portion of the impression is seen sticking up above the rest of the impression. Check it for any obvious bubbles or voids. Small ones should be filled with wax before pouring. Large ones may require a remake of the impression. If there are any obvious undercuts, remove them with a sharp knife or scissors. It will save considerable trouble when the wax pattern is made later.

Fig. 3-23 After a full arch cast has been poured, a removable die should be fabricated. In this case, the cast was mounted in a Di-Lok tray.* This permits the use of a removable die without any possible interference between a dowel pin on the bottom of the die and the dowel-core preparation deep within the die.

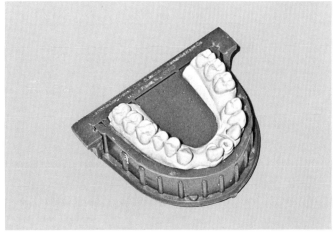

* Di-Lok Tray, Di-Equi Dental Products Distributors Inc., New York, NY.

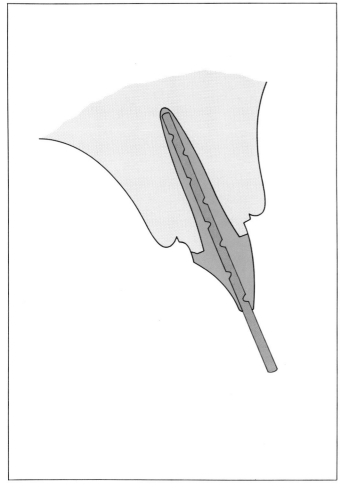

Fig. 3-24 The wax pattern can now be fabricated on the die and working cast.

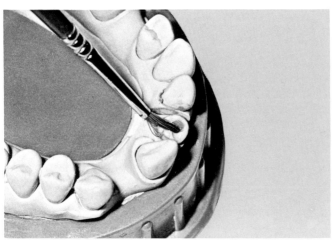

Fig. 3-25 Lubricate the die copiously with a die lubricant.* Make sure that the dowel preparation is well filled.

* Die-Sep, J. F. Jelenko & Co., New Rochelle, NY.

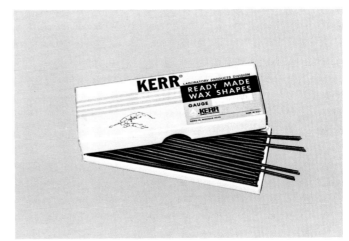

Fig. 3-26 Dead soft, 12 gauge round wax forms* will be used for forming the dowel.

* Ready Made Wax Shapes, Kerr Dental Mfg. Co., Romulus, MI.

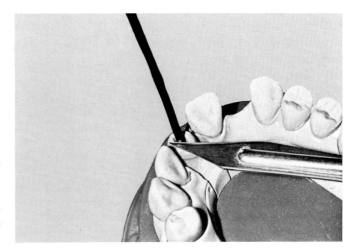

Fig. 3-27 One of the 12 gauge wax sprues is placed into the bottom of the canal in the lubricated die. Cut it off flush with the top of the coronal tooth structure with a sharp laboratory knife.

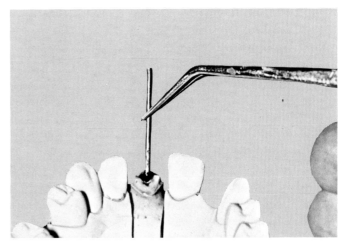

Fig. 3-28 Grasp a piece of wire, such as a straightened paper clip, in cotton pliers and heat it in the flame of a Bunsen burner. Plunge the hot wire into the canal until it touches bottom, melting all the wax in the canal. Hold it steady until the wire cools and the wax solidifies.

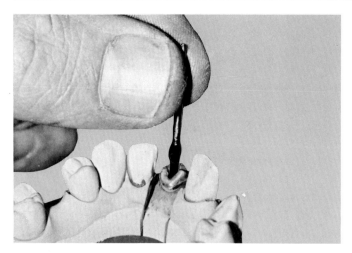

Fig. 3-29 Gently pump the wire and soft wax dowel in and out a few times to make sure that it is easily removable from the die.

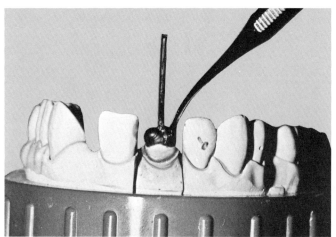

Fig. 3-30 Use regular inlay wax to build up the core portion of the wax pattern.

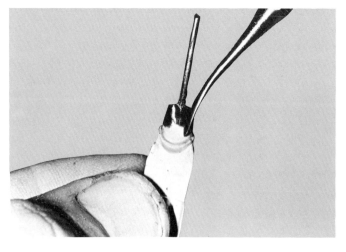

Fig. 3-31 Finish the margins of the core with a warm beaver tail burnisher to produce as well fitting a casting as possible.

Fig. 3-32 The completed wax pattern will have the paper clip protruding from the incisal edge or lingual surface. The wire will serve as the main support of the sprue. Soft wax is added to the wire to thicken it to the diameter of a 10 or 12 gauge sprue.

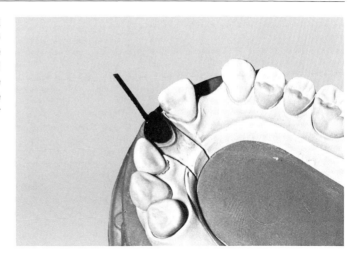

Fig. 3-33 Remove the pattern from the die by grasping the wire-backed sprue and pulling straight off incisally. Insert the wire into the crucible former. Smooth up the wax coating on the wire. The dowel-core pattern should not extend beyond the end of the casting ring. If it does, shorten the wire-backed sprue to place the apical end of the dowel within the confines of the ring.

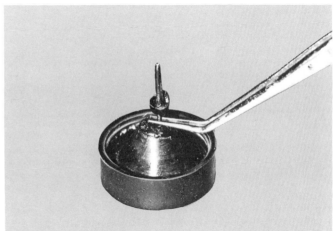

Fig. 3-34 Invest the pattern in gypsum-bonded investment, without asbestos, if the dowel-core will be cast in gold. If the dowel-core will be nickel-chrome, line the ring with a liner that has been thoroughly compressed so that expansion will be decreased or eliminated. The phosphate-bonded investments used for nickel-chrome alloys are difficult to break out without some form of separating liner. The wire in the sprue will be pulled out of the investment, if it doesn't fall out, after burnout and before casting.

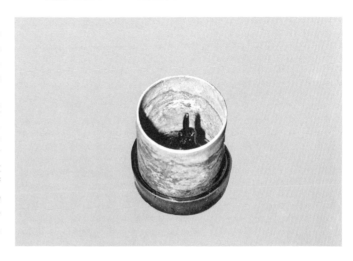

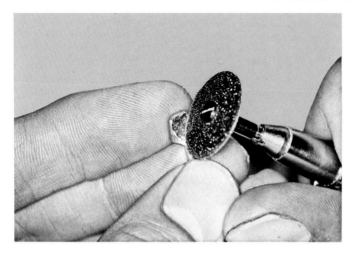

Fig. 3-35 Cut off the sprue attachment and smooth down any gross irregularities on the coronal portion of the dowel-core with a Carborundum separating disc.

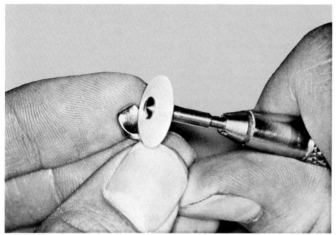

Fig. 3-36 Finish the core to a matte finish with a rubber wheel. Use a coarse, large diameter disc for base metal dowel-cores and a smaller, less abrasive disc for gold alloy castings.

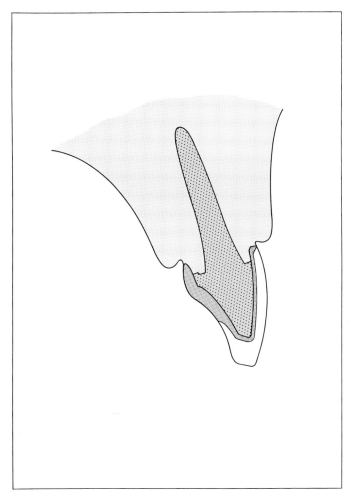

Fig. 3-37 The final crown can be fabricated over the dowel-core seated in the die. If the laboratory procedures are performed meticulously, the restoration can be completed with an even greater savings of chair time by eliminating an appointment for cementation of the dowel-core and making an impression. There is always the risk, however, that a slight discrepancy in fit or the double thickness of cement from seating the dowel-core and crown at one appointment could produce a less than optimum fit.

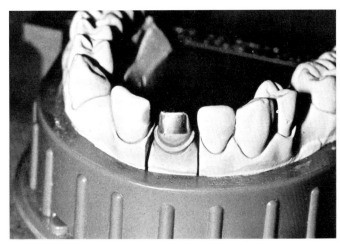

Fig. 3-38 Place the completed dowel-core in the die, making sure that it is completely seated.

91

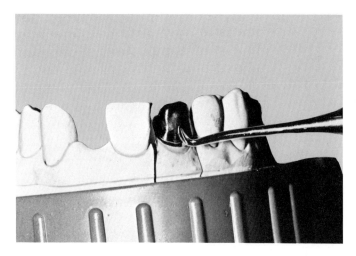

Fig. 3-39 Relubricate the die and lubricate the core. Then wax a coping for the porcelain fused to metal crown.

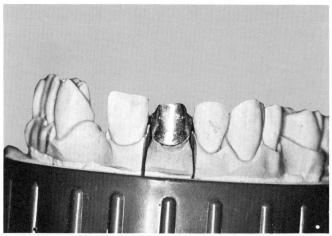

Fig. 3-40 Seat the cast coping back on the dowel-core in the die. The marginal adaptation should be good, and the fit of the coping over the dowel-core and die should be passive, i.e., there should be no binding.

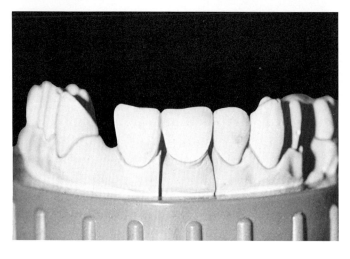

Fig. 3-41 Porcelain is baked to the coping to complete the porcelain fused to metal restoration.

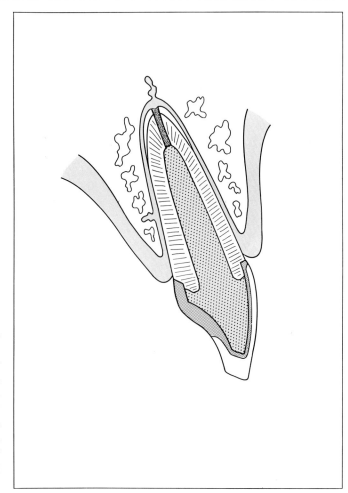

Fig. 3-42 The dowel-core and crown are cemented sequentially, paying particular attention to the marginal fit of the porcelain fused to metal crown. If there is any question about the ability of the technician to produce a well fitting crown with this "non-stop" technique, then the dowel-core should be cemented and an impression made for fabrication of the porcelain fused to metal crown.

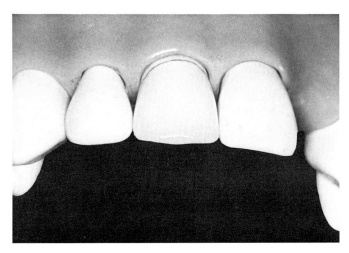

Fig. 3-43 The completion of the endodontic treatment comes with the cementation of the final restoration.

References

1. Dooley, B. S.: Preparation and construction of post-retention crowns for anterior teeth. *Aust Dent J,* 12:544–550, Dec. 1967.

2. Michnick, B. T. and Raskin, R. B.: A multiple post-core technique. *J Prosthet Dent,* 39:622–626, Jun. 1978.

3. Sall, H. D.: Restorative technics for endodontically treated teeth. *Dent Surv,* 53:45–47, Sept. 1977.

4. Baraban, D. J.: The restoration of pulpless teeth. *Dent Clin N Amer,* 12:633–653, Nov. 1967.

5. Fellman, S.: Indirect technic for gold core and crown restoration for non-vital teeth. *Dent Surv,* 40:41–43, Mar. 1964.

6. Baumhammers, A.: Simplified technique for a one-unit cast dowel crown. *Dent Dig,* 68:468–472, Oct. 1962.

7. McLean, J. W.: The alumina tube post crown. *Brit Dent J,* 123:87–92, Jul. 1967.

8. Mazzuchelli, L.: Post and core construction. *R I Dent J,* 5:11–15, Jun. 1972.

9. Burnell, S. C.: Improved cast dowel and base for restoring endodontically treated teeth. *JADA,* 68:39–45, Jan. 1964.

10. Rosenstiel, E.: Impression technique for cast core preparations. *Brit Dent J,* 123:599–600, Dec. 1967.

11. Greenwald, A. S.: Cast gold post and crown restoration. *Dent Surv,* 41:47–50, Apr. 1965.

Chapter 4

Custom Dowel-Core (Two-Piece)

While the single-piece dowel-core is an excellent restoration for anterior teeth and premolars, it is not often used for molars. If a molar has any bulk of coronal tooth structure remaining, it usually will be restored with an amalgam or a composite resin pin core. If there is no remaining coronal tooth structure, it is necessary to use at least one dowel to provide stability against horizontally directed forces. If a molar is to be restored with a single crown, a single-piece cast dowel-core or an amalgam or composite resin core with one or more prefabricated metal dowels can be used. A cast dowel-core placed down one primary canal of a posterior tooth can be successful if the root is fairly long, straight, and bulky.

However, if a severely damaged tooth is to be subjected to the stresses of acting as an abutment for a fixed bridge or removable partial denture, more resistance and retention are required. Because of the root divergence found in most molars, using a dowel-core with two or three parallel dowels extended

into multiple roots can be quite hazardous. Therefore, a multiple-piece dowel-core with separate dowels should be employed.[1-4] The dowel-core for a mandibular molar is usually divided into mesial and distal segments. The maxillary molar dowel-core is composed of facial and lingual components, with the dowels in the two facial canals paralleling each other. When the mesiofacial and distofacial canals are too divergent to permit parallel dowels, a separate third dowel is required.

For a two-piece dowel-core to achieve maximum strength and retention from the dowels in divergent canals, the pieces must be rigidly bound together after insertion. A number of ingenious methods have been proposed for accomplishing this. The core can be made in two halves held together by interlocking lugs[3, 5, 6] which can be formed from a commercially available non-rigid connector pattern or by cutting a keyway or dovetail in one half of the core pattern. Horizontal bolts have also been described for this purpose.[5]

95

A commonly used solution for the problem is the fabrication of a core with an integral dowel and a channel in the core through which an accessory dowel is cemented.[1, 2, 7-10] The hole for the interlocking accessory dowel is aligned with a preparation in another diverging canal. The accessory dowel acts as a dowel-core within a dowel-core, and its divergent direction helps to "nail" the core in place. The secondary dowel can be a prefabricated post or wire, or it can be a cast custom dowel. A variation on this theme uses a core with *no* attached dowel. It is pierced with channels for two or three diverging separate dowels which, when inserted and cemented, will hold the core firmly in position.[5]

Finally, the core can be fabricated in two halves with pin holes in the first half and interlocking pins in the second half.[11, 12] The core is pinned together when both halves have been cemented in the tooth. Any of these interlocking methods can be fabricated by the direct technique,[1, 2, 9, 10, 12] or by the indirect technique.[5-8, 11] All of these methods involve some intricacy, if not outright precision. They can be accomplished far more expeditiously and simply in most cases if the indirect technique is employed.

The method shown on the following pages will be for a two-piece dowel-core utilizing two pins for locking the core together. However, clinical examples will also be shown for dowel-cores bound together by nonrigid connectors and secondary dowels through the core.

Fig. 4-1 A broken-down maxillary first molar is to be used as an abutment for a fixed bridge. The severe destruction from caries, previous restorations, and endodontic access make it a candidate for a two-piece dowel-core.

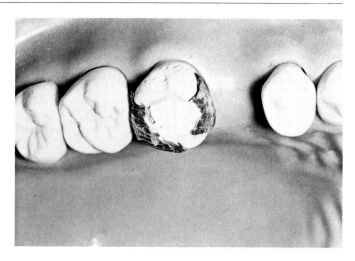

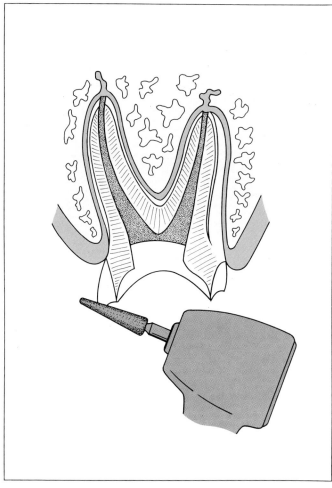

Fig. 4-2 Begin the preparation by removing previous restorations, bases, temporary restorations, caries, and undermined tooth structure.

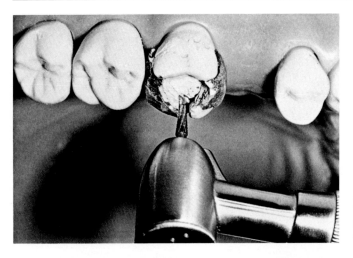

Fig. 4-3 Use a large crosscut fissure bur (No. 702 or No. 558) to remove the amalgam, bases, and temporary restorations.

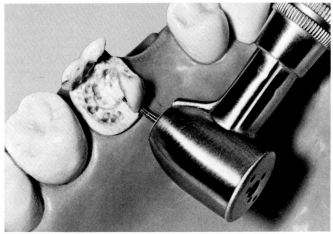

Fig. 4-4 Undermined and unsupported tooth structure must be removed at this time. Preserving it until later can only serve to cloud the true need for retention and resistance of any core that will be placed to support a crown.

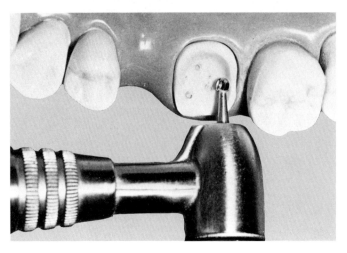

Fig. 4-5 Remove any remaining caries or jagged tooth structure on the root face. The absence of supragingival tooth structure to provide lateral support, and the lack of sound tooth structure around the pulp chamber will dictate the use of a two-piece dowel-core for this bridge abutment.

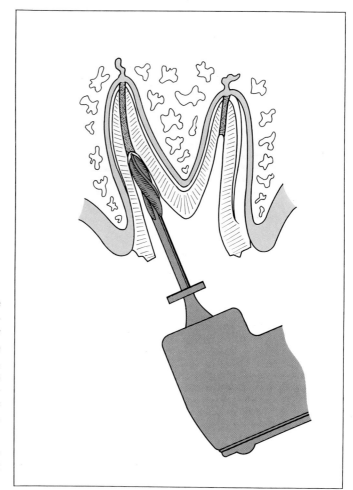

Fig. 4-6 Peeso reamers will be used for preparation of the canals. On the average maxillary molar, the palatal canal will be enlarged to the diameter of a No. 4 reamer, while a No. 3 will be used as the final instrument for the two facial canals. The distal of the average mandibular molar will require a No. 3 Peeso reamer, and the mesial will be instrumented to the width of a No. 2 reamer.

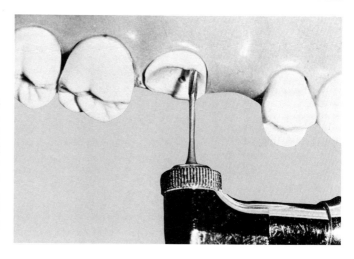

Fig. 4-7 After removing the gutta percha with a hot instrument, enlarge the first facial canal to approximately half its length. It will be the size of a No. 3 reamer on most teeth. Because there will be multiple divergent dowels, their length need not be as great as that required for a single dowel.

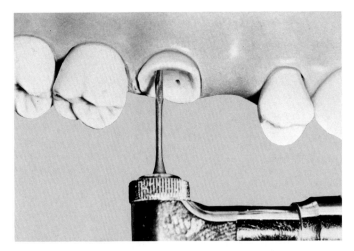

Fig. 4-8 Ream the second facial canal, comparing it frequently with the first facial canal to insure that they are parallel with each other.

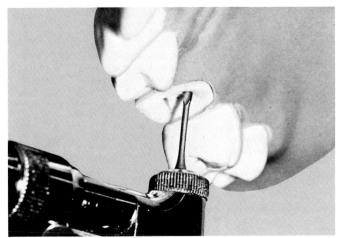

Fig. 4-9 Finally, the palatal canal is prepared. It will not be parallel with the other two canals.

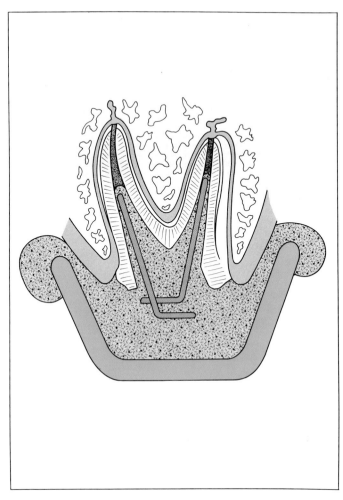

Fig. 4-10 In order to fabricate the dowel-core by the indirect technique, it is important to obtain an accurate impression of the canal preparation. A short segment of wire (paper clip) is placed in each canal to reinforce the impression dowel.

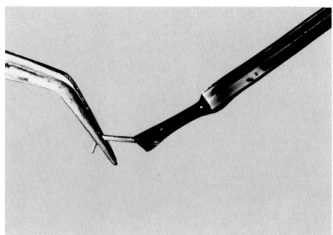

Fig. 4-11 Coat the reinforcing pins or wires with the adhesive for the type of impression material being used.

101

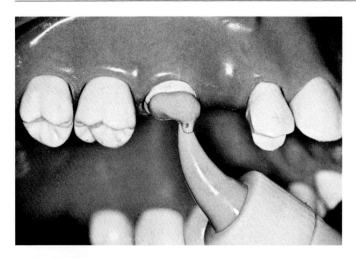

Fig. 4-12 Inject impression material into the pulp chamber area and over the entire root face.

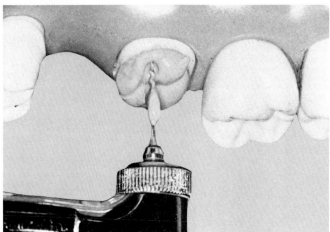

Fig. 4-13 A Lentulo spiral paste filler is placed into each canal to insure that impression material uniformly coats the walls of all of the canals. A light-bodied material of runny consistency works best for this.

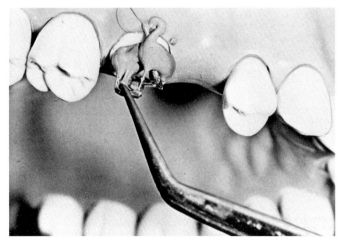

Fig. 4-14 Insert one of the wires or pins into each canal to reinforce the impressions of the dowel preparations.

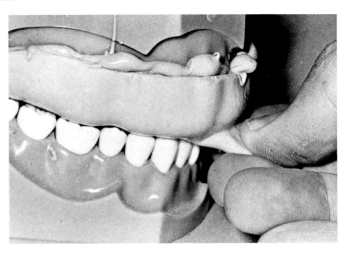

Fig. 4-15 Seat the full arch impression tray. With most elastomeric materials, a more accurate result will be obtained with a custom tray. To remove the tray, pull straight down occlusally until the seal is broken. Then retrieve it from the dowel preparations by moving it occlusal and *slightly* to the facial of the prepared tooth.

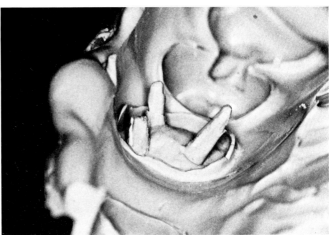

Fig. 4-16 Inspect the impression for complete detail. Make sure that the full length of each dowel preparation has been reproduced, that each dowel is still firmly attached, and that no large voids are present. Small voids can be filled in with soft wax at this time. Any pronounced undercuts on any of the dowels should be removed with sharp tissue scissors.

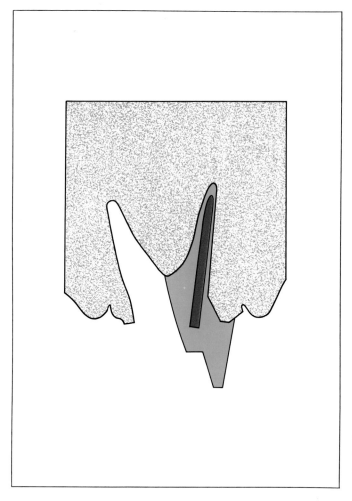

Fig. 4-17 The wax pattern for the facial half of the dowel-core will be fabricated first. On a mandibular tooth, it would be the mesial half.

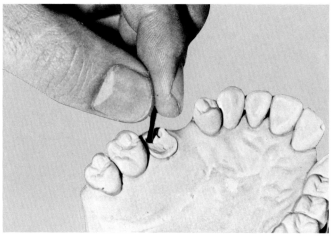

Fig. 4-18 Try 14 gauge solid plastic sprues* into the two facial canals. Trim them with coarse garnet discs so they will fit easily to the bottom of their respective dowel preparations.

* Williams Gold Refining Co., Inc., Buffalo, NY.

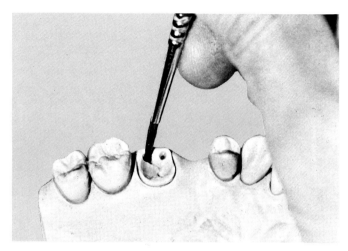

Fig. 4-19 Lubricate the cast thoroughly with a die lubricant.* Place the brush to the bottom of each canal. Wait a few minutes for the lubricant to soak in and apply a second coat.

* Die-Sep, J. F. Jelenko & Co., New Rochelle, NY.

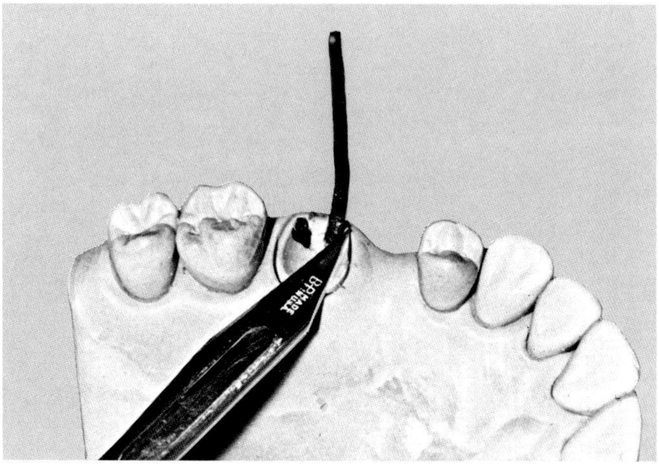

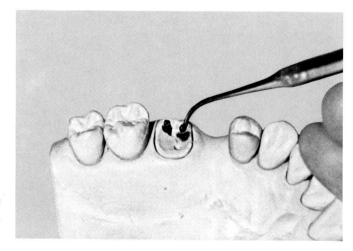

Fig. 4-20 Place soft, round wax forms* into each of the two facial canals. Cut them off flush with the root face of the tooth.

* Ready Made Wax Shapes, Kerr Dental Mfg., Romulus, MI.

Fig. 4-21 Plunge a hot PKT No. 1 instrument to the bottom of each of the canals, melting the soft wax completely.

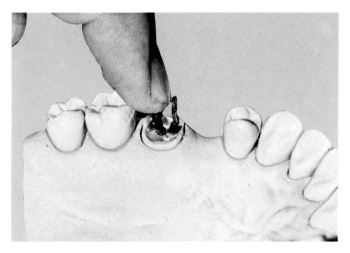

Fig. 4-22 While the wax in the facial canals is still soft, insert the trimmed solid plastic sprues into the wax and shove each of them to the bottom of its respective canal.

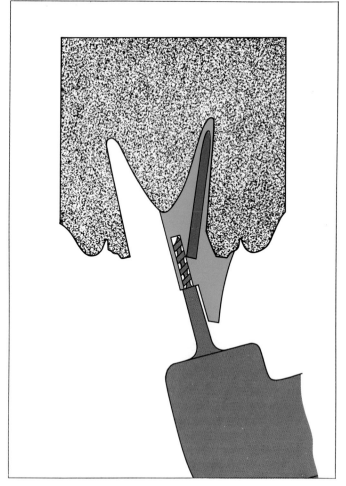

Fig. 4-23 To provide the locking mechanism for tying the two halves of the core together after cementation, pin holes are drilled in the facial half of the core.

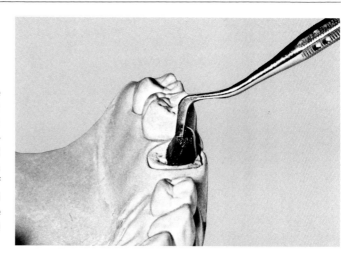

Fig. 4-24 The facial half of a core is produced. Its external axial contours will be consistent with the axial walls of a full crown preparation. The lingual surface will be a flat, smooth surface which parallels the path of insertion of the palatal canal. Use an enamel hatchet to carve a 1.5 mm. wide ledge or shoulder in the occlusal third of the lingual surface.

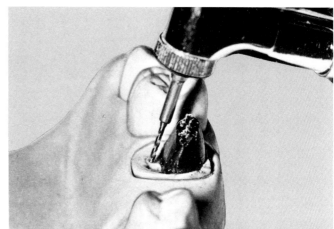

Fig. 4-25 Carefully align a 0.7 mm. drill with the path of insertion of the palatal canal.

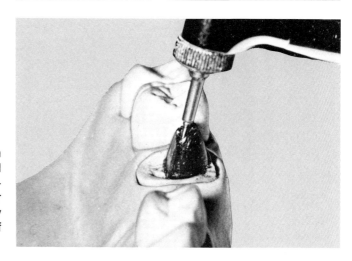

Fig. 4-26 Drill the pin holes in the ledge, making them parallel with each other and the path of insertion of the palatal canal. For maximum effectiveness, they should extend the full length of the core.

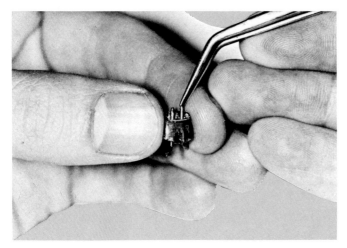

Fig. 4-27 A short section of thin pencil lead (graphite in a Kaolin base) is placed in each pin hole before investing. This will keep the holes patent during burnout and casting. About 2 mm. of graphite should show at each end of the pin hole to insure that the rods will be held securely by the investment. If the graphite fits loosely, use a small bead of sticky wax to tack it to the pattern.

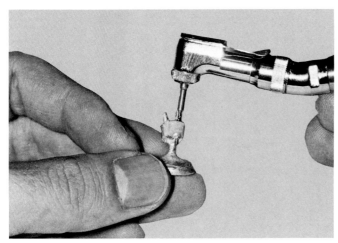

Fig. 4-28 The pattern is invested, burned out, and cast. A gold alloy should definitely be used for this type of dowel-core because graphite (carbon) rods are employed to maintain the pin holes. The contamination of a chromium containing alloy with carbon will increase brittleness and decrease corrosion resistance.[13, 14] Use the 0.7 mm. drill to remove the graphite from the pin holes.

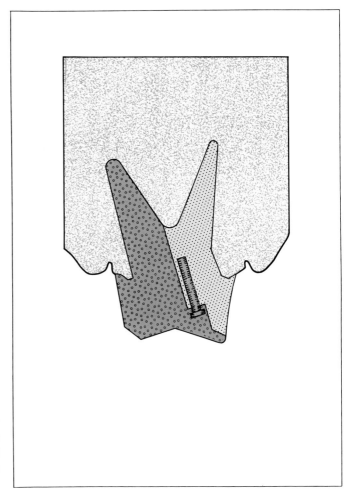

Fig. 4-29 Once the casting for the facial half of the dowel-core has been fabricated, the lingual half can be made against it on the cast.

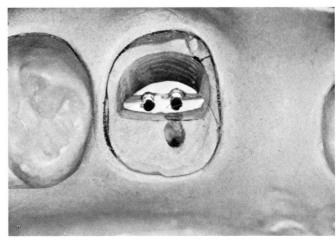

Fig. 4-30 Seat the completed facial of the dowel-core into the facial canals. Check to make sure that the lingual surface and the two pin holes are parallel with the dowel preparation in the palatal canal.

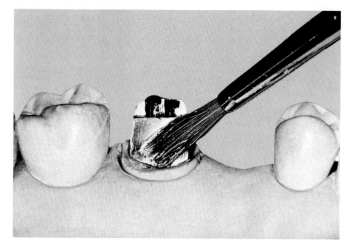

Fig. 4-31 Insert nylon bristles into each of the pin holes and lubricate the lingual surface of the facial core. Relubricate the palatal canal profusely.

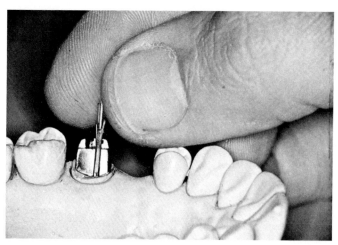

Fig. 4-32 Try a 14 gauge plastic sprue into the palatal canal. Trim the sides of the sprue with a coarse garnet disk to allow the sprue to slip easily to the bottom of the canal.

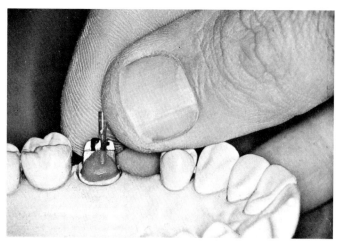

Fig. 4-33 Although wax could be used for the pattern for the lingual half of the core, acrylic resin* is shown here. Acrylic forms a hard surface that cannot be distorted by manipulation. A more precise fit, which is essential for post cementation rigidity, will be possible. A fresh mix of resin is placed in the mouth of the canal, and the trimmed plastic sprue is seated to place.

* Duralay, Reliance Dental Mfg., Chicago, IL.

Fig. 4-34 When the acrylic is near polymerization, pump the sprue in and out several times to insure that it will not lock into any undercuts.

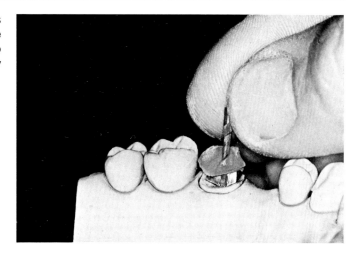

Fig. 4-35 Use a second mix of acrylic to build-up the required bulk for the lingual half of the core. Be sure that the acrylic is especially well adapted against the flat lingual surface of the facial half of the core. The resin should surround the nylon bristles projecting from the facial core, and it should overlay the occlusal aspect of the facial core.

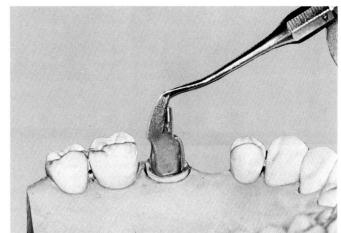

Fig. 4-36 Use garnet discs and carbide burs to shape the axial contours and occlusal planes of the lingual core. The core should now resemble a tooth preparation for a full crown.

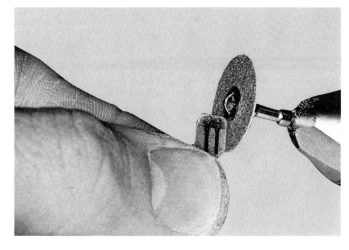

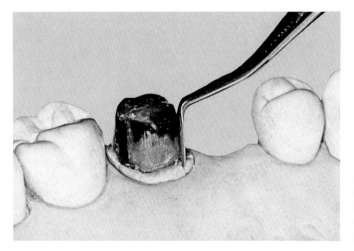

Fig. 4-37 Use inlay wax to touch up any voids in the acrylic pattern. Margins should be well adapted, and axial surfaces should be free of undercuts.

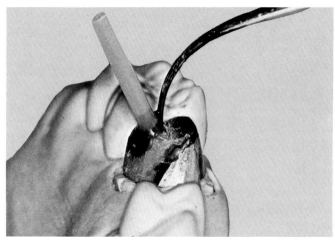

Fig. 4-38 A 10 gauge hollow plastic sprue is attached with sticky wax to the mesio-lingual cusp tip at the angle shown. Withdraw the lingual half of the pattern, invest it in a gypsum-bonded investment, burn it out, and cast it in a Type III or IV gold alloy.

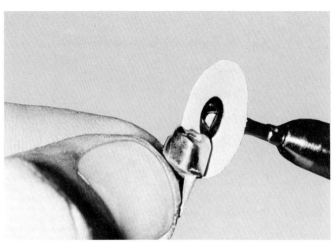

Fig. 4-39 After retrieving the casting from the ring, finish the axial surfaces with abrasive discs and rubber wheels.

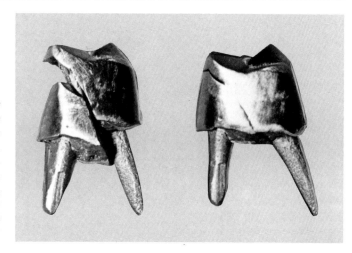

Fig. 4-40 The lingual half of the core is positioned occlusal to the facial half so the pins can be inserted into the pin holes (left). The two halves are brought together (right). If the two halves do not fit together as completely as shown here, check for small nodules of gold or remnants of investment in the line angles.

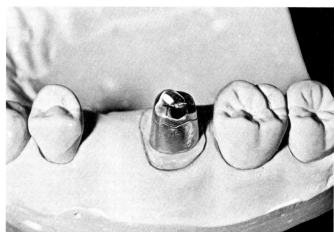

Fig. 4-41 The two halves of the dowel-core are assembled on the working cast to insure that they will fit together in the tooth.

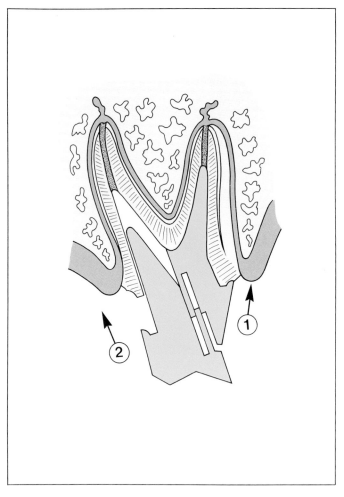

Fig. 4-42 The two-piece dowel-core is now ready to be cemented in the tooth to rebuild it for placement of the final restoration. The facial half will be cemented first (1), followed immediately by the lingual half (2). On a mandibular tooth the mesial would be first, followed by the distal.

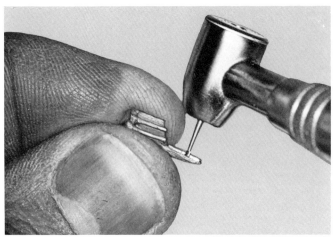

Fig. 4-43 Cut a v-shaped cement vent down the length of each dowel to assist complete seating and the prevention of damaging stresses.

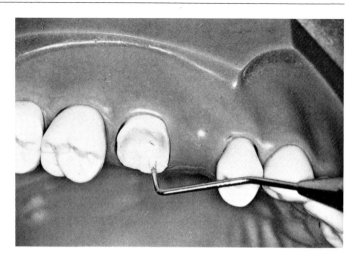

Fig. 4-44 Mix zinc phosphate to a thin consistency and apply it to the dowel preparations and the pulp chamber area. While a Lentulo spiral is preferred for coating the walls of the canals, a periodontal probe can be used if a Lentulo instrument is not available.

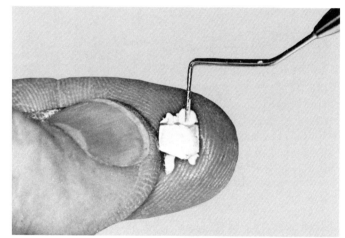

Fig. 4-45 Coat the dowels of the facial half of the dowel-core. Use a Lentulo spiral or a periodontal probe to get cement into the pin holes.

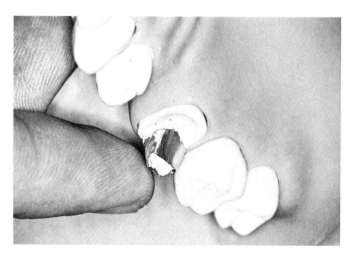

Fig. 4-46 Cement the facial dowel-core using only finger pressure to seat the dowel-core completely.

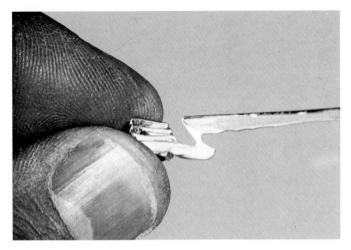

Fig. 4-47 Coat the dowel on the lingual half of the dowel-core with zinc phosphate cement. Make sure that the pins have also been completely coated with the cement.

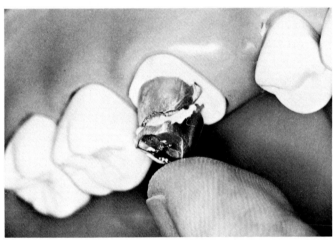

Fig. 4-48 Seat the lingual half of the core, taking care to insert the pins into the pin holes. The palatal dowel will fit into the canal.

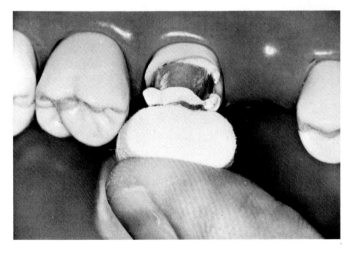

Fig. 4-49 Exert steady pressure on the dowel-core with a cotton roll. Wipe off any cement which has extruded around the periphery of the dowel-core or from between the two parts. Avoid wooden sticks, malleting, or any other technique which would have a tendency to develop stress in the tooth.

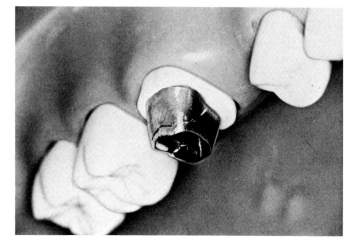

Fig. 4-50 The cemented dowel-core is now ready for completion. The finish line is touched up with a chamfer diamond to provide space for a bulk of metal adjacent to the acute margin in the final crown.

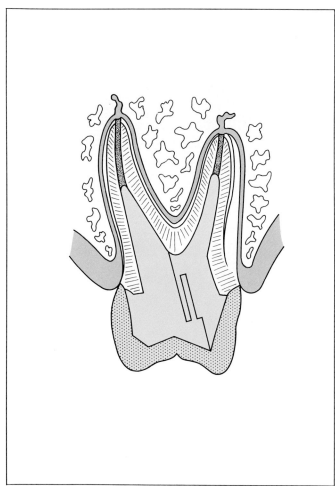

Fig. 4-51 With the two-piece dowel-core cemented in place, the tooth is ready for fabrication of the final restoration. The margin of the final restoration will be placed on solid tooth structure to provide a marginal seal and to provide a band of reinforcing metal apical to the core.

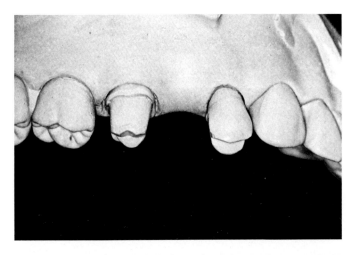

Fig. 4-52 On the working cast, the molar with the dowel-core looks as any other molar with a full veneer preparation would.

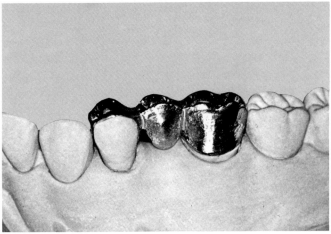

Fig. 4-53 The framework for the porcelain fused to metal bridge is shown, with a partial veneer retainer on the premolar.

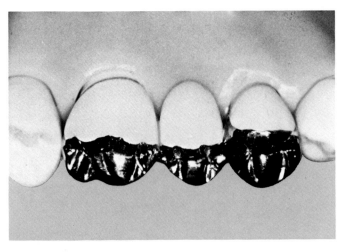

Fig. 4-54 The completed bridge is cemented in the mouth.

Fig. 4-55 The middle or pier abutment for a five unit bridge had to be restored with a two-piece dowel-core before the bridge could be fabricated. Loss of the abutment tooth would have made it necessary to place a long span bridge from first premolar to third molar, or resort to a removable partial denture. Neither alternative was considered desirable for this patient. The cement line can be seen between the facial and lingual halves.

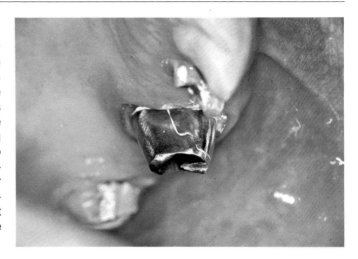

Fig. 4-56 A box form was placed in the distal of the dowel-core during fabrication. This accommodated the nonrigid connector that would be placed in the distal aspect of the retainer on this pier abutment.

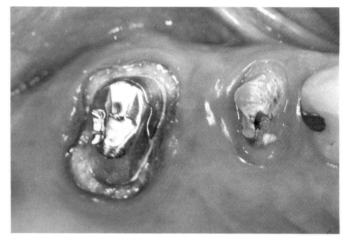

Fig. 4-57 The completed bridge is seen after cementation, extending from first premolar to first molar to third molar. There is a nonrigid connector between the second molar pontic and the first molar retainer.

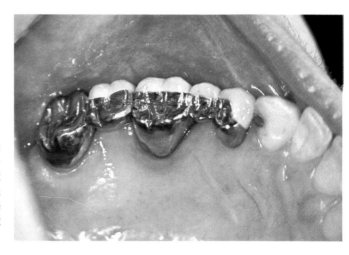

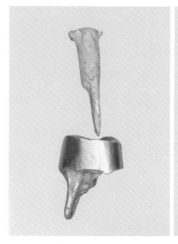
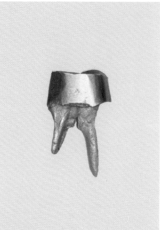

Fig. 4-58 This two-piece dowel-core consists of a core which is firmly attached to the two facial dowels and a separate palatal dowel with a slightly tapered core and orientation lugs (left). When the secondary dowel-core is slipped through the primary core, the divergent dowels will provide excellent retention (right).

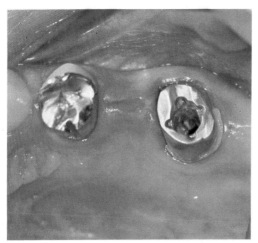

Fig. 4-59 The primary core, attached to the facial dowels, is shown in position on the tooth prior to cementation. The four keyways are evident around the orifice of the channel for the secondary dowel-core.

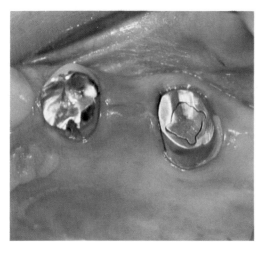

Fig. 4-60 The palatal dowel-core is seen inserted through the facial dowel, with the orifice lugs in the keyways.

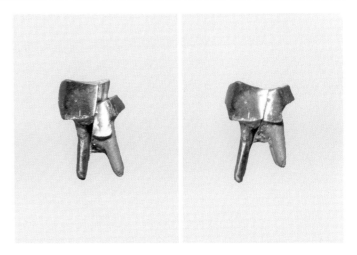

Fig. 4-61 This dowel-core is held together by a precision attachment.* The male segment of the attachment, which is part of the palatal dowel and core, is inserted into the female part of the attachment in the lingual surface of the facial portion of the dowel-core (left). When the palatal portion is pushed down, the two halves of the dowel-core are rigidly connected (right).

* P-D Attachment, Howmedica Inc., Chicago, IL.

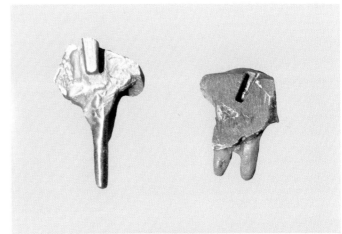

Fig. 4-62 The key, on the facial aspect of the palatal half of the dowel-core, and the keyway in the facial half must be aligned with the palatal dowel.

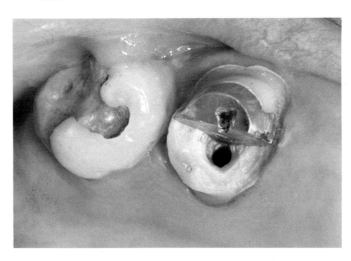

Fig. 4-63 The facial half of the dowel-core is shown in position on the tooth. The alignment of the palatal canal and the keyway is clearly evident in this photograph.

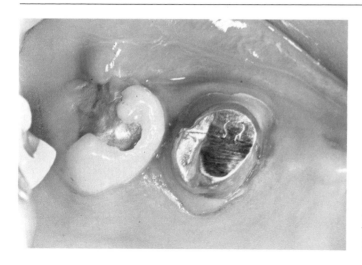

Fig. 4-64 The lingual half of the dowel-core is slipped into position with the key firmly seating into the keyway.

References

1. Bangs, S. A.: Non-parallel cast post core. *Dent Surv,* 54:48–50, Jan. 1978.

2. Lovdahl, P. E. and Dumont, T. D.: A dowel-core technique for multirooted teeth. *J Prosthet Dent,* 27:44–47, Jan. 1972.

3. Perel, M. L. and Muroff, F. I.: Clinical criteria for posts and cores. *J Prosthet Dent,* 28:405–411, Oct. 1972.

4. Spangler, C. C.: Posts and cores: Some new ideas. *Dent Surv,* 56:33–35, Jun. 1980.

5. Henry, P. J. and Bower, R. C.: Post core systems in crown and bridgework. *Aust Dent J,* 22:46–52, Feb. 1977.

6. Rosen, H.: Operative procedures on multilated endodontically treated teeth. *J Prosthet Dent,* 11:973–986, Sept. 1961.

7. Lister, A. E.: A post crown for molars with divergent roots. *Brit Dent J,* 133:161, Aug. 1972.

8. Michnick, B. T. and Raskin, R. B.: A multiple post-core technique. *J Prosthet Dent,* 39:622–626, Jun. 1978.

9. Wearn, D. I.: Posts and cores in divergent canals. *Aust Dent J,* 19:346–348, Oct. 1974.

10. Welsh, S. L. and Priddy, W. L.: Direct fabrication of interlocking endodontic posts. *J Prosthet Dent,* 39:115–117, Jan. 1978.

11. Abdullah, S. I. and Bjorndal, A. M.: A cast gold base for endodontically treated molar roots where divergent form precludes parallel post construction. *Dent Dig,* 76:187–189, Apr. 1970.

12. Shillingburg, H. T., Roane, J. B. and Wilson, K. R.: Two-piece dowel-cores for endodontically treated molars. *CDS Rev,* 71:23–27, Nov. 1978.

13. Duncanson, M. G.: Nonprecious metal alloys for fixed restorative dentistry. *Dent Clin N Amer,* 20:423–433, Apr. 1976.

14. Phillips, R. W.: *Skinner's Science of Dental Materials,* 7th ed. Philadelphia: W. B. Saunders Co., 1973, p. 644.

Chapter 5

Dowel-Core Under a Crown

There are occasions when a tooth which has been restored with a crown will fracture, causing the displacement of the crown. This is caused by weakened structural integrity of the crown as a result of previous restorations, caries, small diameter of coronal tooth structure, brittleness, trauma, or a combination of some or all of these factors. Such a tooth may have been endodontically treated without placement of a dowel-core, or it may still have been vital.

Very often the fracture of the tooth will mean remaking the crown, or, in severe cases in which the fracture extends too far apically, it may even mean loss of the tooth. There are conditions which may permit much less drastic treatment, however. Crowns that meet two criteria can be reused. First, the fracture must be restricted to coronal tooth structure without extending far enough apically to intersect the finish line. Second, the crown must exhibit adequate margins and have acceptable contours and esthetics.

The tooth is restored endodontically if that has not already been done. A dowel preparation is then made in the canal, and a dowel-core is fabricated using the inside of the crown as a matrix for the coronal portion of the dowel-core pattern.

Several different ways of accomplishing this end have been described. Custom cast dowel-cores have been used extensively for this purpose, with patterns made entirely of acrylic resin[1-4] or wax.[5, 6] A combination pattern has been described in which the dowel is wax and the core is acrylic.[7] A similar technique uses a wax core with a precision plastic dowel.[8] An alternate approach, popular because it can be accomplished in a single appointment, uses a composite resin core built around a stainless steel prefabricated dowel[8, 9] or orthodontic wire.[10] A cut-off silver point has been described for an emergency temporary repair.[11]

The technique shown in this chapter will

123

be that for the custom dowel-core made with an acrylic resin pattern. With minor alterations involving the fabrication of the dowel, the same technique could be employed in fabricating dowel-cores with precision plastic dowel patterns.

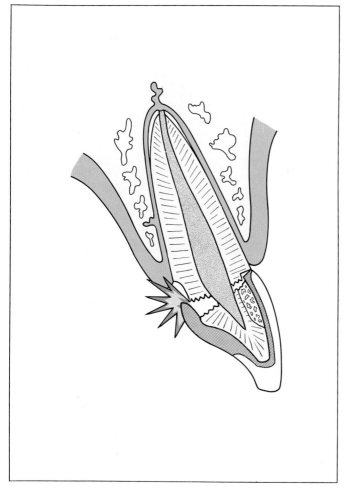

Fig. 5-1 The fracturing of coronal tooth structure under a crown can be very distressing to the patient. It could make useless an otherwise good prosthetic appliance, such as a bridge or a removable partial denture, which might rely on the tooth as an abutment.

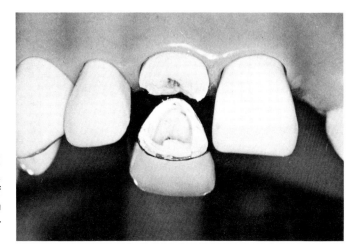

Fig. 5-2 The crown is separated from the maxillary central incisor. Examination reveals the cause of the failure: the coronal tooth structure has fractured off completely.

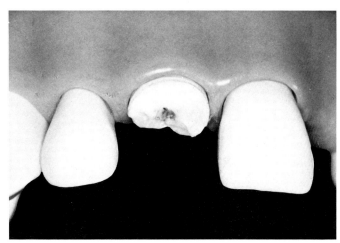

Fig. 5-3 Examination of the tooth reveals an almost total absence of coronal tooth structure. A dowel-core is obviously needed.

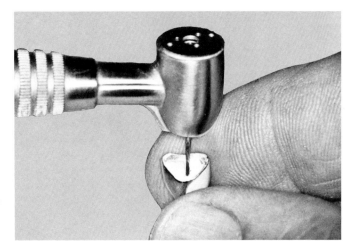

Fig. 5-4 Use a high speed bur initially to remove the bulk of cement and tooth structure remaining in the crown.

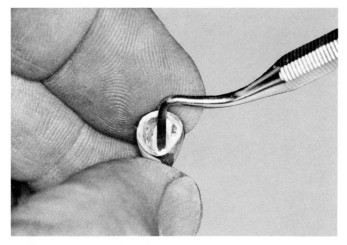

Fig. 5-5 Change to a large, sharp spoon excavator to remove any clinging particles of cement. A bur should not be used at this point because it could nick the inner surface of the crown, producing undercuts that would interfere with the seating of the crown on the core.

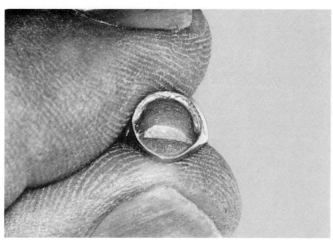

Fig. 5-6 Inspect the inside of the crown to be sure that no cement remains anywhere. Look for rough areas and undercuts that would interfere with seating of the dowel-core. It may be necessary to smooth the irregularities with a carbide nondentate tapered fissure bur.

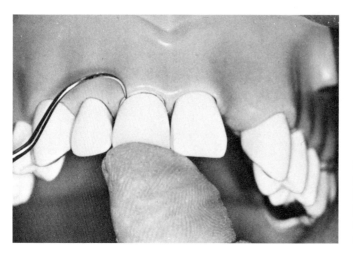

Fig. 5-7 Place the crown back on the stub of the tooth preparation. While holding the crown firmly in place, check the margins very carefully to insure good adaptation.

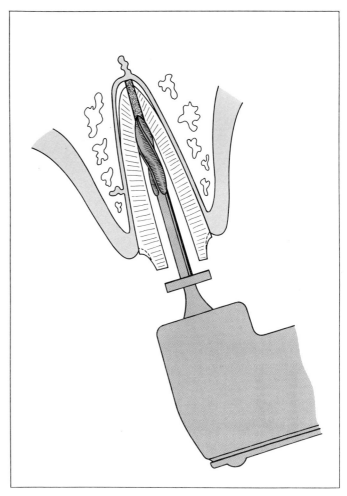

Fig. 5-8 After endodontic treatment, the dowel space is prepared with a Peeso reamer. This instrument is chosen because its non-cutting tip will follow the cleared canal, or the soft gutta percha.

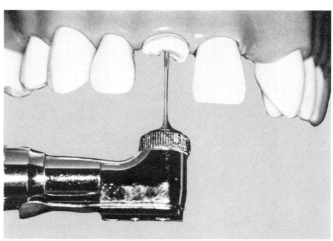

Fig. 5-9 Remove as much gutta percha as possible with a hot instrument before starting the dowel preparation. Use the largest reamer which will fit into the canal. A radiograph can be utilized to verify the dowel preparation length so that necessary adjustments can be made.

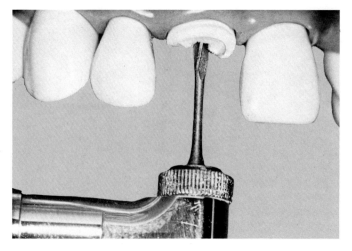

Fig. 5-10 Use the series of graduated reamer sizes to progressively enlarge the canal to the size selected for the tooth being restored.

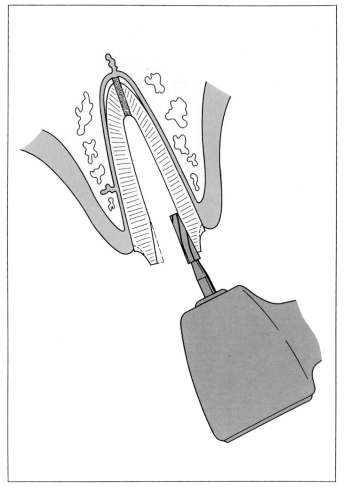

Fig. 5-11 The need for anti-rotational stability in this type of restoration is great because there is little or no coronal tooth structure remaining. One or two vertical grooves are placed in the walls of the canal to serve as keyways to orient the final dowel-core.

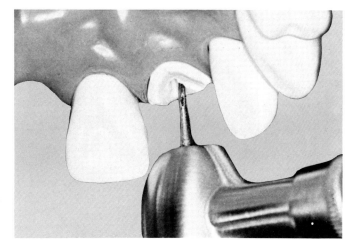

Fig. 5-12 The keyway is made the length of the cutting blade of a No. 170 bur. Its depth is the diameter of the bur, and it is placed in the area of greatest bulk of tooth structure. A second one is added only on larger teeth.

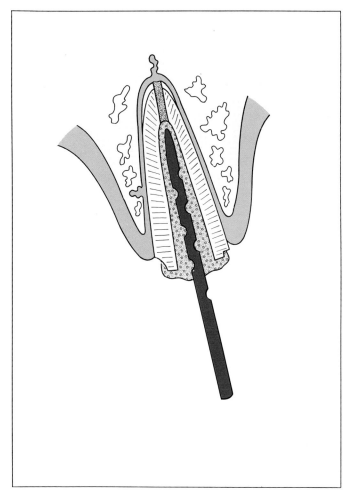

Fig. 5-13 A dowel is fabricated of a solid plastic sprue and acrylic resin.* No effort is made to fabricate the core at this time.

* Duralay, Reliance Dental Mfg. Co., Chicago, IL.

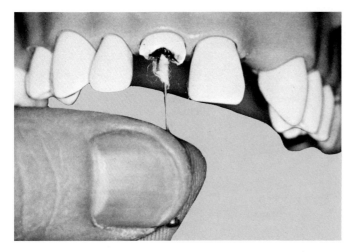

Fig. 5-14 Wrap a cotton pellet around a No. 1 Peeso reamer and dip it into Duralay lubricant. Insert the reamer with lubricant into the canal and pump it to make sure the entire canal is well coated.

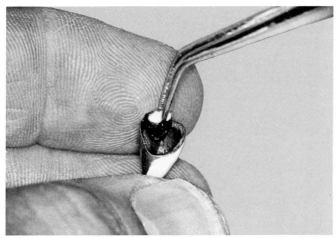

Fig. 5-15 Use a large cotton pellet to apply copious amounts of lubricant to the inside of the crown.

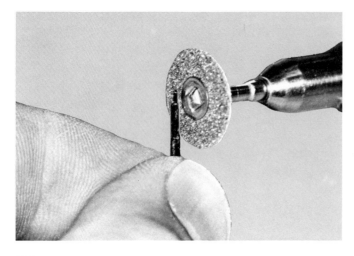

Fig. 5-16 Trim a 14 gauge hard plastic sprue* with a garnet disc so that it can slip easily all the way into the canal.

* Williams Gold Refining Co., Inc., Buffalo, NY.

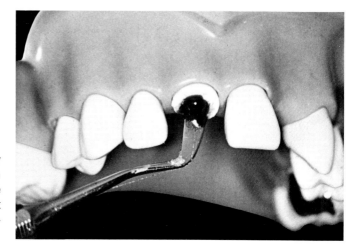

Fig. 5-17 Prepare a thin runny mix of Duralay and place as much as possible in the mouth of the lubricated canal with the flat blade of a plastic filling instrument.

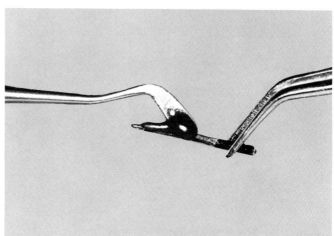

Fig. 5-18 Coat the trimmed plastic sprue with monomer and then cover it with Duralay.

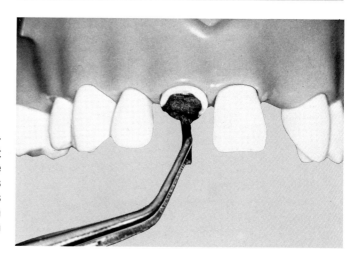

Fig. 5-19 Insert the resin covered sprue in the canal until it touches the apical end of the preparation. Wipe off any excess that extends onto the root face, as this material could interfere with the complete seating of the crown later.

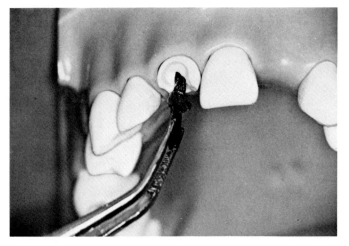

Fig. 5-20 When the resin around the sprue becomes doughy, grasp the sprue sticking out of the tooth and pump it up and down several times. This will prevent the pattern from being locked into the canal.

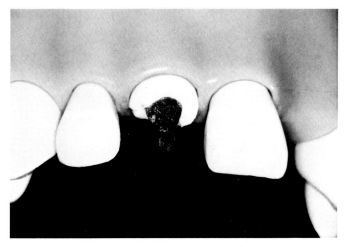

Fig. 5-21 Trim any remaining excess acrylic around the dowel which might interfere with the crown's complete seating. Shorten the dowel so that it also will not interfere with the crown.

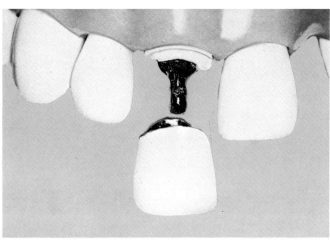

Fig. 5-22 Try the crown over the dowel to make sure that the dowel and Duralay flash have been trimmed sufficiently to permit complete seating of the crown.

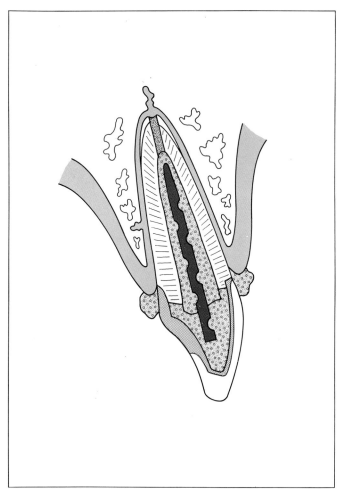

Fig. 5-23 The crown, lubricated and filled with acrylic resin, is placed over the dowel and remnants of the crown preparation. The coronal portion of the dowel-core is fashioned in this way, with the crown serving as a matrix.

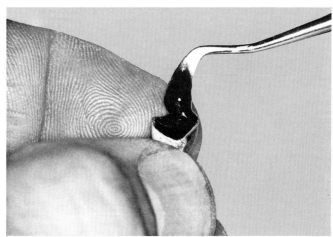

Fig. 5-24 Fill the lubricated crown to the margins with a fresh thin mix of Duralay.

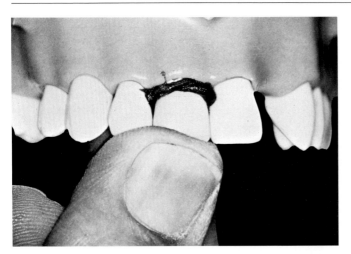

Fig. 5-25 Place the resin-filled crown over the stump of the crown preparation and seat it forcefully. Check its alignment with the adjacent teeth.

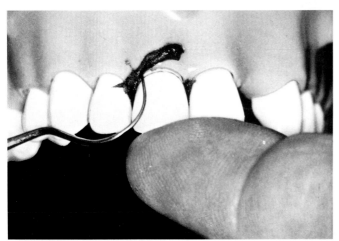

Fig. 5-26 The acrylic around the margins is scraped away and the margins are checked with a sharp explorer to confirm complete seating.

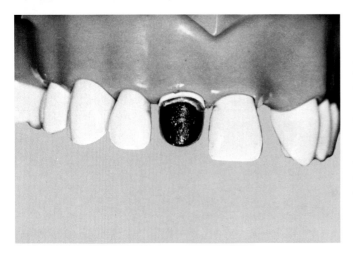

Fig. 5-27 When the acrylic has achieved a tough, doughy consistency, remove the crown from the preparation. The acrylic will have been molded into the shape of a crown preparation by the inside of the crown. After scraping the flash from the margins, lift the polymerizing dowel-core from the preparation several times to prevent its locking into any undercuts. Reseat it and then replace the crown to complete the curing process.

Fig. 5-28 After the acrylic has polymerized, remove the dowel-core from the tooth and trim away any remaining excess around the margins. Smooth all external surfaces of the coronal portion with rubber wheels. Fill in any voids with soft wax. Reseat the dowel-core for a final check.

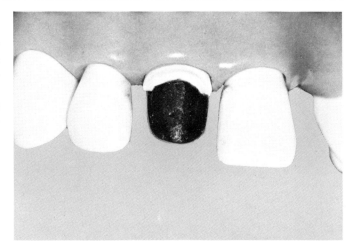

Fig. 5-29 A lingual view of the completed dowel-core pattern.

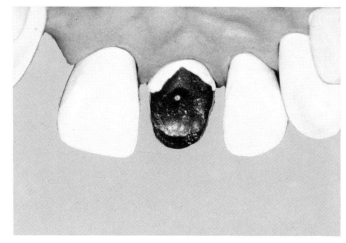

Fig. 5-30 The sprue is attached to the pattern in the middle of the lingual surface. The attachment must *not* blend into the linguo-proximal or incisolingual line angles. Their presence will aid in trimming the sprue attachment site later. If the casting is to be of nickel-chrome, invest the pattern in phosphate-bonded investment.* If the dowel-core is to be cast in gold alloy, use gypsum-bonded investment.**

 * High Temp, Whip Mix Corporation, Louisville, KY.
** Beauty-Cast, Whip Mix Corporation, Louisville, KY.

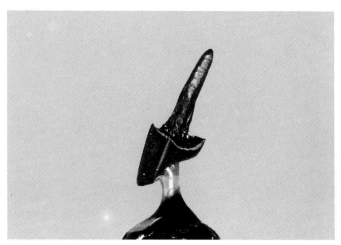

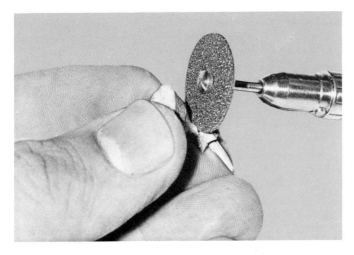

Fig. 5-31   After the casting has been made and retrieved from the investment, the sprue is removed with a separating disc.

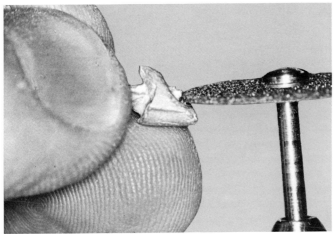

Fig. 5-32   The sprue attachment area is ground smooth with a separating disc, taking care to blend it into the surrounding contours of the lingual surface. The presence of the line angles and a little of the lingual surface around the sprue attachment make this task much simpler.

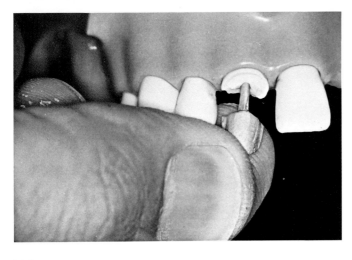

Fig. 5-33   The dowel-core is tried in to verify the fit of the casting.

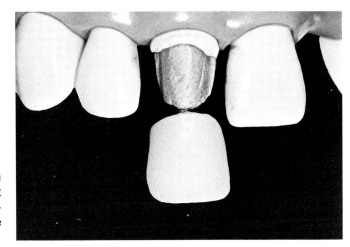

Fig. 5-34 The crown is tried in over the dowel-core to insure that no casting irregularities will prevent complete seating of the crown over the dowel-core.

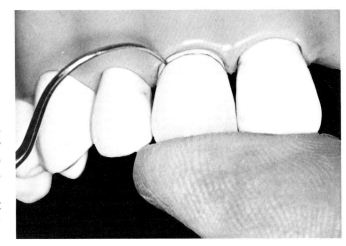

Fig. 5-35 Hold the crown securely in position and carefully check the margin with a sharp explorer to verify complete seating. After the crown has been removed, clean all the lubricant from its inner walls using cotton pellets and acetone.

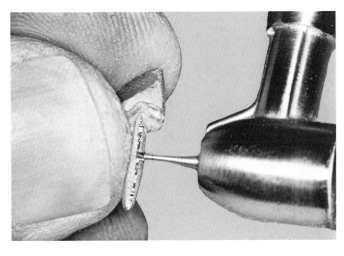

Fig. 5-36 A v-shaped cement escape vent is placed on the side of the dowel with a No. 34 carbide bur. By allowing easy escape of the cement from the hydraulic chamber formed by the dowel in the canal, lateral stresses should be diminished greatly during cementation.

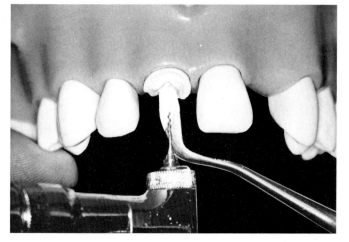

Fig. 5-37 Cover the blade of a plastic instrument with a thin mix of zinc phosphate cement and hold it lingual and incisal to the mouth of the prepared canal. Use a slowly rotating Lentulo spiral paste filler to carry the cement into the canal and coat its walls. Add more cement until the canal appears to be filled.

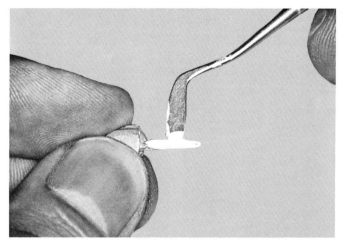

Fig. 5-38 Coat the dowel with cement and insert it into the canal.

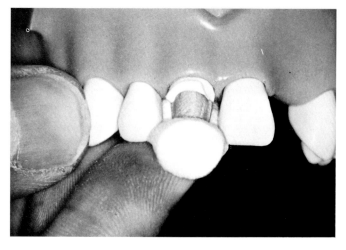

Fig. 5-39 Place a cotton roll over the incisal edge of the dowel-core and seat it with slow, steady finger pressure. This will allow the cement to escape ahead of the dowel.

Fig. 5-40 While the dowel is being inserted in place by the dentist, the assistant should coat the inner surfaces of the crown with zinc phosphate. Once the dowel is in place, immediately seat the crown over it using firm finger pressure. Once again, check the margins carefully with a sharp explorer to verify complete seating. Check the occlusion while the cement is still soft.

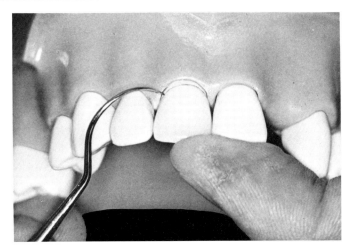

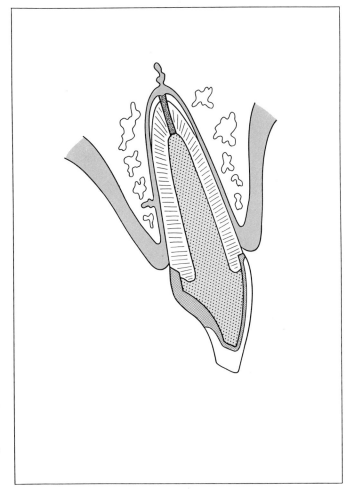

Fig. 5-41 The use of a dowel-core fabricated after the crown makes it possible to save the crown on a fractured tooth. It will have the same strength and retention it would have had if the dowel-core had been placed before the crown was made.

139

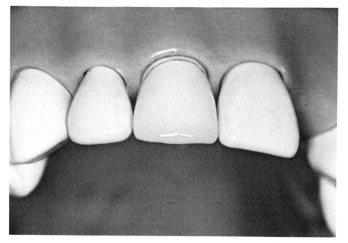

Fig. 5-42 The crown cemented over the dowel-core is returned to full function. This technique should be regarded only as a repair measure. The reader should be cautioned against relying on it to the extent that teeth needing dowel-cores will not receive them before crowns are placed in the errant belief that "If it breaks, *then* we'll do the dowel-core." The time and place of fracture cannot be controlled, nor can its extent. The crown or even the tooth might be lost as a result.

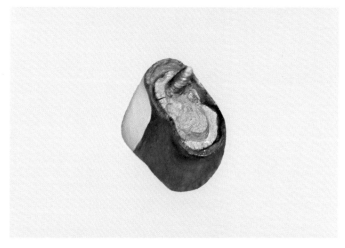

Fig. 5-43 This maxillary premolar had been built-up with an amalgam core and a tapered threaded dowel before the crown was fabricated. The core had failed.

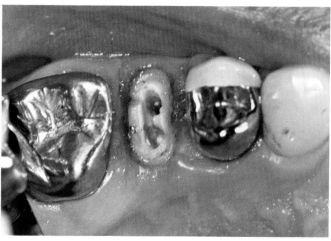

Fig. 5-44 There was no coronal tooth structure to retain the crown. A dowel-core build-up was required.

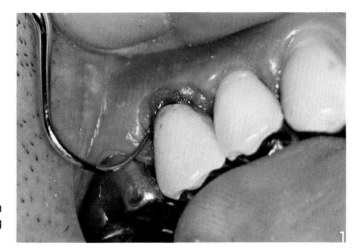

Fig. 5-45 The crown is shown in position while the core was being formed.

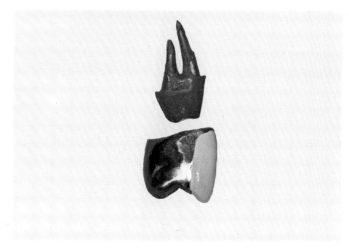

Fig. 5-46 The crown and the dowel-core pattern are shown after they were removed from the tooth and flash had been removed from the dowel-core.

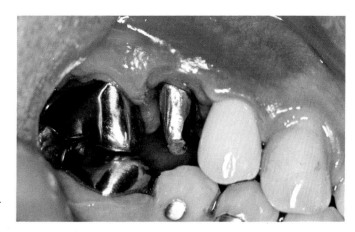

Fig. 5-47 The completed dowel-core is seen in the tooth.

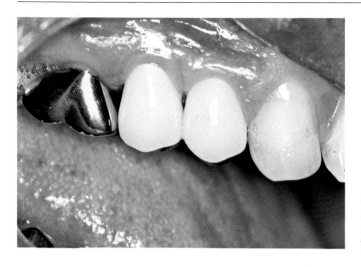

Fig. 5-48 The crown, cemented over the new dowel-core, is shown five months after cementation.

References

1. Asawa, G. N.: Cast dowel-core fabrication on a pre-existing crown. *Dent Surv,* 48:36–37, Jan. 1972.

2. Goldrich, N.: Construction of posts for teeth with existing restorations. *J. Prosthet Dent,* 23:173–176, Feb. 1970.

3. Priest, G. and Goerig, A.: Post and core fabrication beneath an existing crown. *J Prosthet Dent,* 42:645–648, Dec. 1979.

4. Tebrock, O. C.: Technique for post-core removal from a crown and a new post-core fabrication. *J Prosthet Dent,* 43:463–466, Apr. 1980.

5. Beheshti, N.: Fabricating a post and core to fit an existing crown. *J Prosthet Dent,* 42:236–239, Aug. 1979.

6. Richardson, J. T. and Padgett, J. G.: Repair technique for a fractured, crowned anterior tooth. *J Prosthet Dent,* 31:409–410, Apr. 1974.

7. Shirdel, K., Azarmehr, P. and Raoufi, M.: Construction of a post and core to fit a completed restoration. *J Prosthet Dent,* 38:229–231, Aug. 1977.

8. Henry, P. J. and Bower, R. C.: Secondary intention post and core. *Aust Dent J,* 22:128–131, Apr. 1977.

9. Federick, D. R.: An application of the dowel and composite resin core technique. *J Prosthet Dent,* 34:420–424, Oct. 1974.

10. Richardson, J. T. and Sox, J. T.: Repair technique for a fractured, crowned tooth. *J Prosthet Dent,* 37:547–549, May 1977.

11. Harris, W. E.: A single-visit endodontic/post crown procedure. *J Ga Dent Assoc,* 45:14–18, Autumn 1971.

Chapter 6

Dowel-Inlay Crown Repair

Teeth that have been restored with crowns will sometimes require endodontic treatment later. It is a good idea to minimize these situations by never placing a cast restoration on a tooth with a pulp cap over an exposure. Nevertheless, not every pulpal complication can be foreseen, and endodontic treatment will occasionally be required after the tooth has been restored.

In most cases, the root canal treatment will be done through the cast restoration. While it is possible to remove a crown, the crown or the tooth preparation under it may be damaged in the process. If an otherwise sound restoration must be penetrated to provide an endodontic access, how will the tooth be restored after the endodontic procedure has been completed?

It is not enough to place an amalgam or composite resin restoration in the access opening for a single-rooted tooth. The tooth structure covered by a crown suffers from the same weakness that besets an endodontically treated tooth before placement of a crown: there is very little left to provide resistance. In fact, the problem is probably a little worse in this case. An endodontic access through a crown is often larger because the crown obscures the morphology of the tooth and makes it more difficult to locate the pulp chamber.

Solutions for this problem have included cast dowels with an attached inlay to close the access opening,[1-3] a prefabricated dowel with a composite resin closure restoration,[4] and a prefabricated dowel with an amalgam seal.[3] This repair process has been referred to as a "secondary intention" dowel[4] or post[3] and core.

If a dowel with an attached inlay is utilized, the inlay is locked to the dowel, and some retention is imparted to the restoration, as well as resistance to laterally directed forces. Because this restoration is a combination of a dowel and an inlay, consistent nomenclature would suggest the use of *dowel-inlay* to describe it.

143

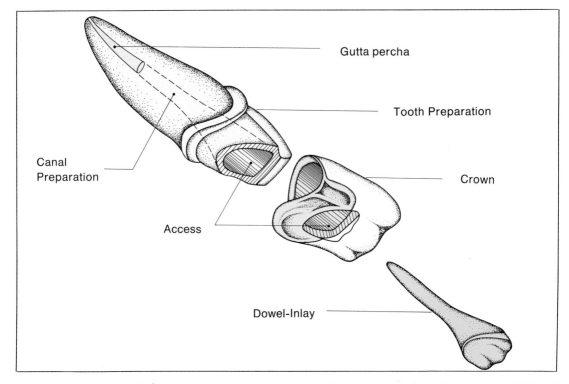

Fig. 6-1   This exploded view shows an endodontically treated tooth with a crown which will be restored with a dowel-inlay. The components are shown separately for clarity's sake: the crown is not removed to fabricate the restoration. (Adapted from Federick and Serene.[4])

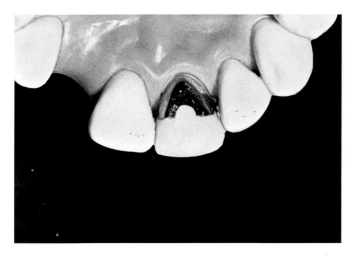

Fig. 6-2   A crown with no other flaws can still see many years of service if some restoration is added to bolster the weakened preparation after the endodontic access has been cut.

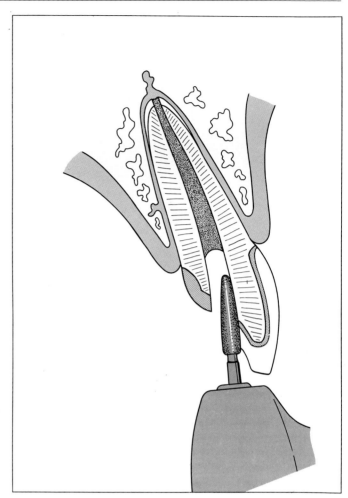

Fig. 6-3 The mouth of the canal must be extended enough to remove any undercuts, particularly toward the facial wall of the preparation. Smooth internal walls are also important to the fit of the inlay component of the restoration.

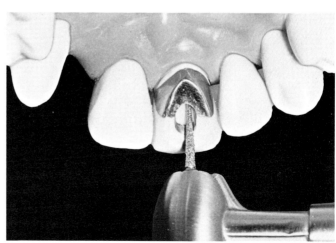

Fig. 6-4 Begin the widening of the orifice of the canal with a round-end tapered diamond. It is especially effective in cutting through any porcelain which may lie on the periphery of the preparation.

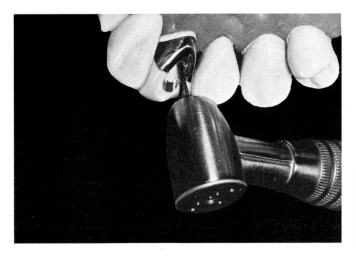

Fig. 6-5 Flare out the incisal 2–3 mm. of the orifice to form the inlay portion of the preparation. Use a No. 170 bur to plane the walls smooth.

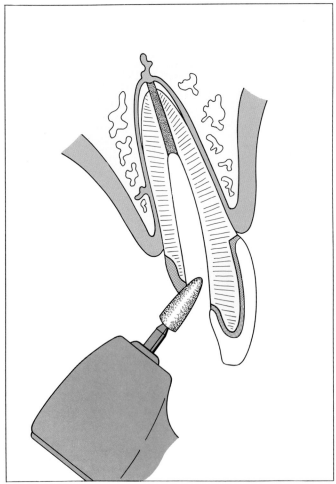

Fig. 6-6 To achieve the best possible marginal adaptation of the final restoration, place a well defined wide bevel (1.0 mm. or greater) around the entire periphery of the mouth of the canal.

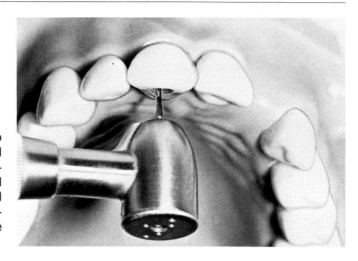

Fig. 6-7 Use a No. 170 bur to form those portions of the bevel which will be placed in un-veneered metal on the lingual surface of the crown. The gingival portion of the bevel will be at approximately a 90° angle to the path of insertion of the dowel.

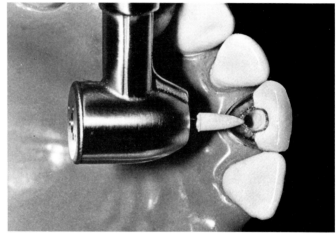

Fig. 6-8 Finishing touches are added to the bevel with a white polishing stone. Because the lingual surface of the crown closely approximates the path of insertion of the dowel, the finish line for the incisal segment of the bevel may not be as well defined.

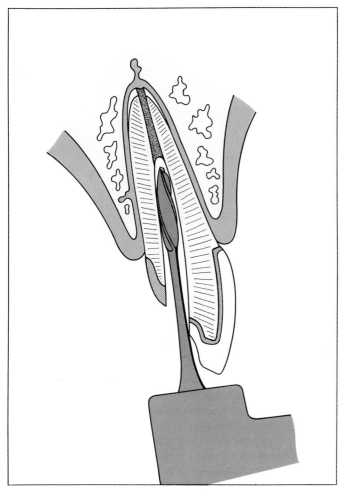

Fig. 6-9 Gates Glidden drills and Peeso reamers will be used for enlarging the dowel space. The canal preparation may be somewhat more curved to the lingual because the incisal edge of the crown stands in the way. The Gates Glidden drill is better for starting this preparation because of its flexible shaft. It can help straighten the canal by cutting away the blocking tooth structure on the lingual aspect of the canal at or slightly apical to the level of the cemento-enamel junction. If a rigid Peeso reamer is used initially, the tip may be forced facially in the apical third of the dowel, causing another and worse undercut.

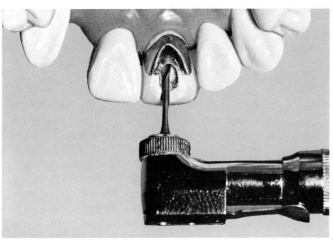

Fig. 6-10 The gutta percha is removed with a hot instrument before starting with the largest Gates Glidden drill that will slip into the canal. Work on the lingual aspect 3–4 mm. apical to the mouth of the canal. Reinstrument the dowel preparation with a Peeso reamer to achieve as straight walls as possible. Use the same diameters recommended for a dowel-core.

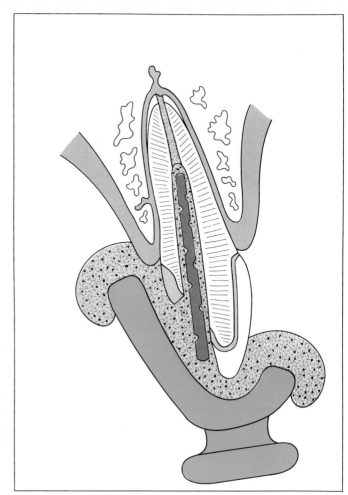

Fig. 6-11 An impression is made of the finished dowel preparation for the indirect fabrication of a dowel-inlay pattern. The indirect technique is chosen primarily because it is easier to manipulate around any undercuts in the canal with an indirect pattern. Any elastomeric material with a reasonably light-bodied injection material can be used.

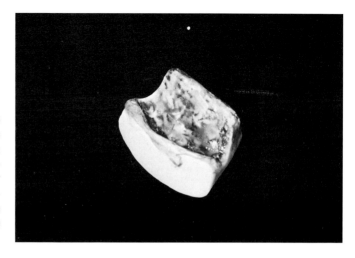

Fig. 6-12 The impression tray is made of tray acrylic and has rests on the incisal edge of the tooth on either side of the tooth being restored. It need extend no farther mesiodistally. Because the impression must draw slightly to the lingual when it is removed, the tray is open on the facial.

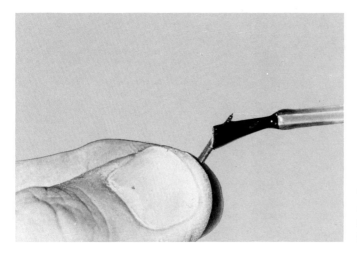

Fig. 6-13 Coat the wire reinforcement for the dowel (a piece
of paper clip) with the specific
adhesive recommended for the
impression material being used.

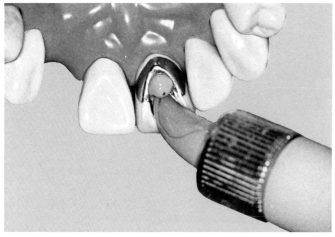

Fig. 6-14 Inject impression
material into the orifice of the
canal. Any material can be used,
but the more elastic light-bodied
silicones are preferable because
of their ease of manipulation.

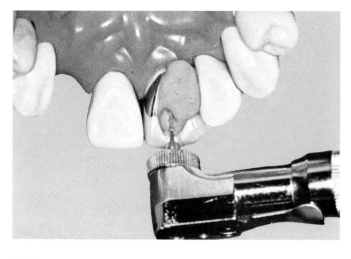

Fig. 6-15 A Lentulo spiral
cement filler is placed into the
canal to thoroughly coat the walls
of the dowel preparation with impression material.

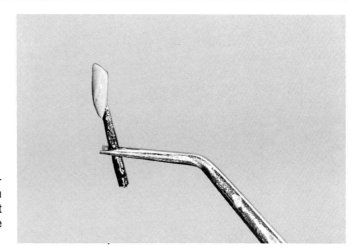

Fig. 6-16 Dip the adhesive-coated wire into impression material on the pad and insert it into the canal. It should protrude at least 2.0 mm. from the canal.

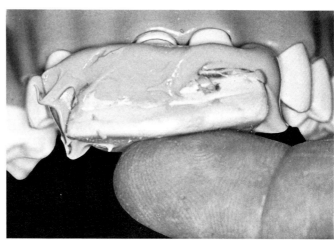

Fig. 6-17 Place the small impression tray over the tooth being restored until it rests firmly on the incisal edges of the teeth. Steady the tray by holding it until the impression material has set.

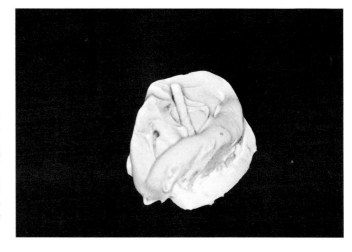

Fig. 6-18 Remove the tray incisally, rolling it slightly to the lingual as you do. Inspect the impression for completeness. Look for undercuts, in the form of bulges, on the sides of the dowel. Remove the more pronounced ones with sharp scissors to simplify fabrication of the dowel-inlay wax pattern.

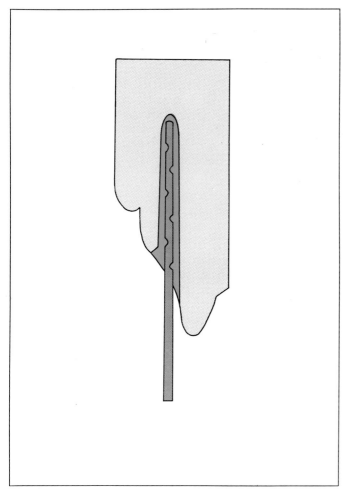

Fig. 6-19 The wax pattern can be fabricated on the die made from the impression of the prepared tooth.

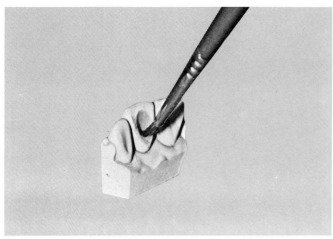

Fig. 6-20 Brush the die thoroughly with a die lubricant.* The dowel preparation should be filled completely.

* Die-Sep, J. F. Jelenko & Co., New Rochelle, NY.

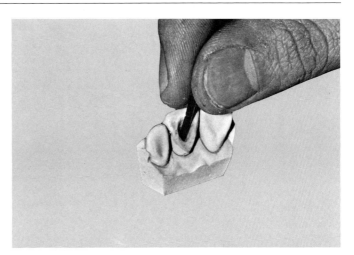

Fig. 6-21 Use dead soft 12 gauge wax forms* for fabricating the pattern of the dowel. Insert one of the wax forms into the canal until it touches bottom. Cut it off flush with the lingual surface of the die with a sharp laboratory knife.

* Ready Made Wax Shapes, Kerr Dental Mfg. Co., Romulus, MI.

Fig. 6-22 Use cotton pliers to hold a piece of wire, made from a shortened paper clip, in the flame of a Bunsen burner. Quickly place the hot wire into the dowel preparation, melting all the soft wax in the canal. Steady the wire until it cools, and the wax solidifies.

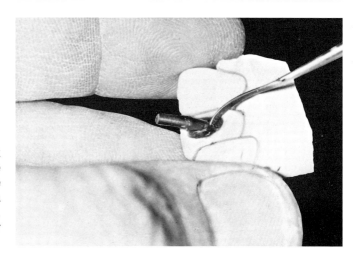

Fig. 6-23 Add the soft blue wax around the wire to fill in the entire dowel space. The margins are smoothed and adapted with a warm instrument with dull edges, such as a beavertail burnisher or a DPT No. 6.

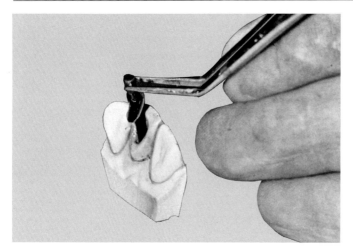

Fig. 6-24 Remove the wax pattern by grasping the wire with cotton pliers. The soft wax should be smeared by minute undercuts in the canal.

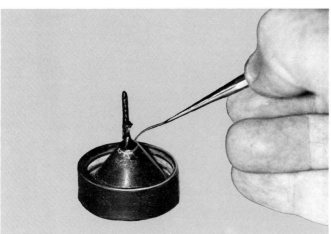

Fig. 6-25 Attach the end of the wire to the crucible former with sticky wax. Make sure that all of the wire brace is covered by some form of wax. The sprue with its wax coating should be about 2.0 mm. in diameter.

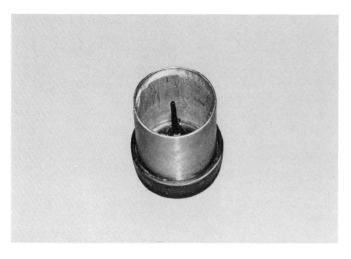

Fig. 6-26 The sprued wax pattern is ready for investing when the ring is in place. No liner is used, if the investment will be gypsum-bonded, for a gold casting. A gold alloy is important for this type of restoration because of the need for good marginal adaptation.

Fig. 6-27 After the wax pattern has burned out, remove the ring from the furnace with casting tongs. Use cotton pliers to extract the paper clip from the middle of the sprue to allow free access of the alloy to the mold.

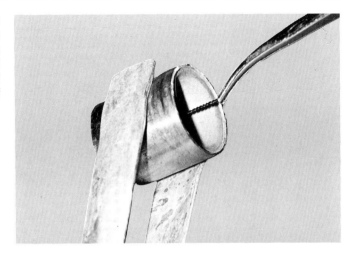

Fig. 6-28 After retrieving the cast dowel-inlay from the investment, clean and pickle it. Try it in the die to check its fit.

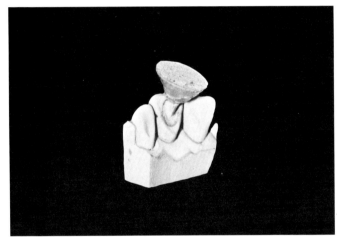

Fig. 6-29 Sprues and buttons are usually removed before a casting is tried in to prevent the application of leverage that is possible with such a large handle on a small dowel. In this situation, however, the button remains attached because it provides the only means of holding the dowel during try-in. Therefore, it must be handled very carefully when the dowel is seated. Be especially careful not to twist it, and not to allow the patient to close on it. Check the margins carefully for adaptation.

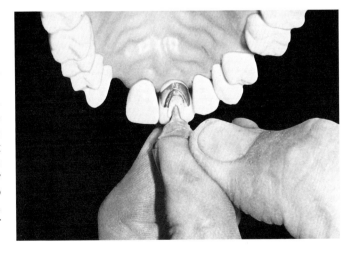

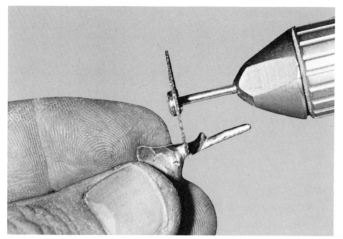

Fig. 6-30 Remove the sprue with a Carborundum separating disc. Trim off the excess contour where the sprue was attached, producing a slight concavity in the lingual surface of the inlay. There should be a v-shaped cement escape vent on the side of the dowel, but it should end about 2.0 mm. from the inlay margin to avoid the possibility of a marginal defect.

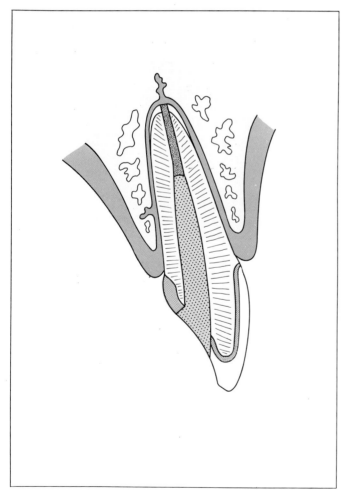

Fig. 6-31 The dowel-inlay is cemented in the canal, providing a closure of the endodontic access and reinforcement of the root and coronal tooth structure under the crown.

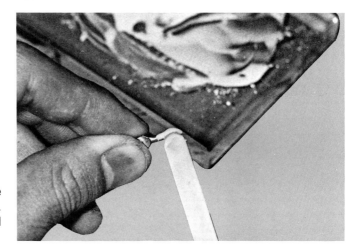

Fig. 6-32 Mix zinc phosphate cement to a thin consistency. Apply it to the dowel, covering all of the surfaces.

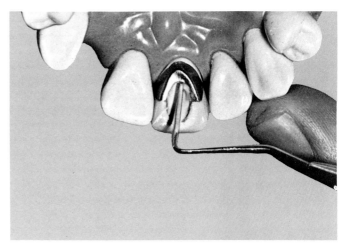

Fig. 6-33 Apply cement to the dowel preparation with a periodontal probe or a Lentulo spiral cement filler. Take care to coat the walls of the canal all the way to the apical end of the dowel preparation.

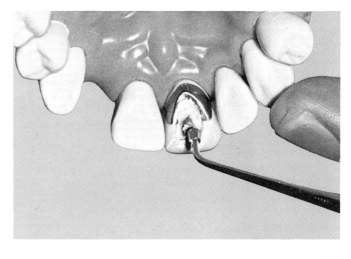

Fig. 6-34 Insert the dowel-inlay into the cement-filled orifice of the canal, pushing it in with finger pressure. Use a condenser to seat the dowel-inlay completely to place. Check the margins with an explorer. Keep pressure on the dowel-inlay with the instrument until the cement has set.

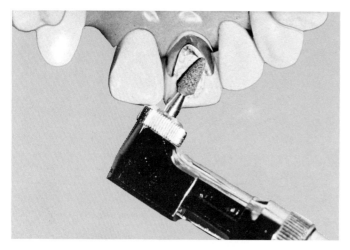

Fig. 6-35 Use a Carborundum stone* to adjust the contour of the dowel-inlay to blend in with that of the adjacent lingual surface. Initial steps can be taken in margin finishing, always orienting the stone so that it revolves from inlay to surrounding crown.

* FL 2 Dura–Green Stone, Shofu Dental Corp., Menlo Park, CA.

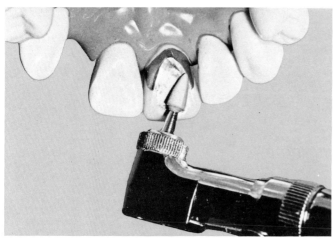

Fig. 6-36 Complete the margin finishing using a white polishing stone* and petrolatum, moving the stone from inlay to crown.

* FL 2 Dura–White Stone, Shofu Dental Corp., Menlo Park, CA.

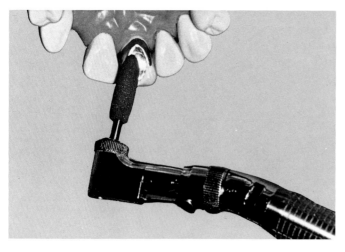

Fig. 6-37 A large, coarse, red rubber point* is used to smooth the surface of the inlay to eliminate scratches produced by the abrasive stones.

* PC 2 Brownie Point, Shofu Dental Corp., Menlo Park, CA.

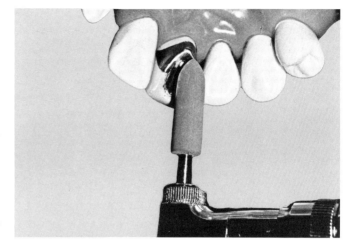

Fig. 6-38 A final polish is added by using a large, fine, green rubber point.*

* PC 2 Greenie Point, Shofu Dental Corp., Menlo Park, CA.

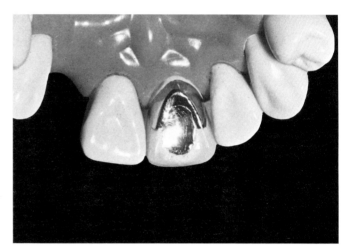

Fig. 6-39 The completed dowel-inlay is seen cemented through a porcelain fused to metal crown.

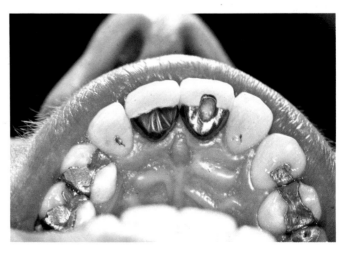

Fig. 6-40 Endodontic treatment became necessary 14 months after insertion of the porcelain fused to metal crown. Following completion of the root canal treatment, a dowel-inlay preparation was made in the tooth.

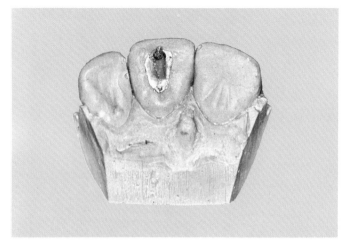

Fig. 6-41 The dowel-inlay, with part of the sprue attached, is tried in the die to verify the fit.

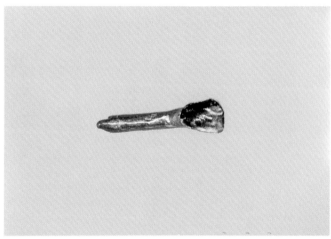

Fig. 6-42 The dowel-inlay is seen before cementation. Notice the concave lingual surface of the inlay component.

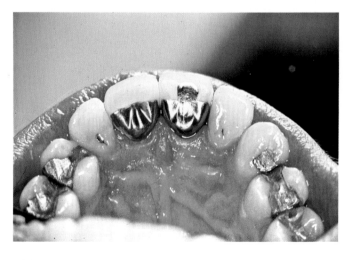

Fig. 6-43 The completed dowel-inlay is cemented in the endodontic access opening in the lingual surface of the porcelain fused to metal crown.

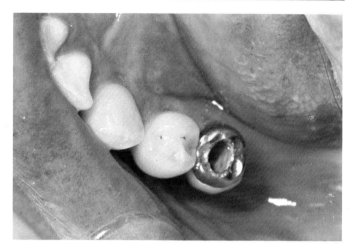

Fig. 6-44 This premolar, which is an abutment for a removable partial denture, has been restored with a crown. It required endodontic treatment later. Because of the stress placed on it and the amount of coronal tooth structure destroyed, a dowel-inlay preparation was made.

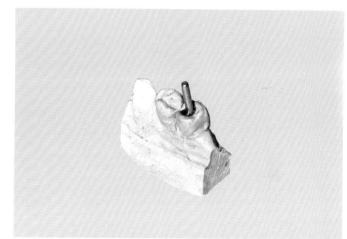

Fig. 6-45 A metal rod, in this case a trimmed bur, was used to reinforce the wax pattern in the die.

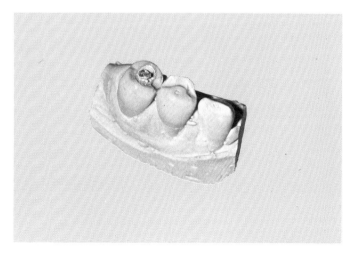

Fig. 6-46 The casting is tried into the die to check its fit. The sprue and button have been removed.

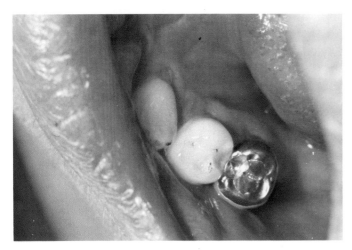

Fig. 6-47 The fully restored tooth is shown after cementation of the dowel-inlay. The inlay segment of the restoration contains a portion of a rest preparation for a removable partial denture.

References

1. Frank, A. L.: Protective coronal coverage of pulpless teeth. *JADA,* 59:895–900, Nov. 1959.

2. Abdullah, S. I., Mohammed, H. and Thayer, K. E.: Restoration of endodontically treated teeth. A review. *J Canad Dent Assoc,* 40:300–303, Apr. 1974.

3. Henry, P. J. and Bower, R. C.: Secondary intention post and core. *Aust Dent J,* 22:128–131, Apr. 1977.

4. Federick, D. R. and Serene, T. P.: Secondary intention dowel and core. *J Prosthet Dent,* 34:41–47, Jul. 1975.

Chapter 7

Precision Parallel Plastic Dowel

The prefabricated precision dowel forms part of a system in which the dowel is designed to fit a canal space shaped by a specific instrument of matching size and configuration. This differs from the custom dowel-core because the canal is prepared to fit the dowel rather than a pattern being made as an impression of the internal aspect of the tooth. The resulting fit may not be as exact,[1] but it is usually clinically acceptable.

Precision plastic dowels are available in parallel and tapered configurations. Parallel dowels exhibit superior retention: studies have found them to be 1.9 times,[1] 3.3 times,[2] and 4.5 times[3] as retentive as prefabricated tapered dowels of equal length. If the surface is serrated, retention will be improved even more.[1]

There is a prefabricated precision dowel pattern which combines a serrated surface with a parallel-sided geometry.* It was designed to be used with one or more parallel pins set in dentin periph-

* Para-Post, Whaledent International, New York, NY

eral to the canal. The pins act primarily as antirotational features, although they may add some retention and resistance to dowel-cores which are lacking those qualities because of tooth size or morphology. The Para-Post is manufactured with a groove running its entire length to act as a cement vent.

Conditions which permit the use of a serrated parallel plastic dowel pattern include a fairly bulky root and a canal which is essentially straight. Because a parallel dowel does not follow the natural taper of most roots, it may not be possible to choose a pattern and drill for every tooth. The dowel picked must be large enough in diameter to include the coronal portion of the canal, but small enough to leave an adequate thickness of dentin at the apical end. If the coronal portion of the canal has been enlarged excessively, a small dowel may fit too loosely, and a larger dowel may cause insufficient tooth structure to be left in the apical section.[1]

In considering a tooth for restoration with this system, it is also necessary to evaluate the tooth structure available for pin placement. If there is insufficient bulk to accommodate pins, keyways can be prepared in the walls of the canals.[4]

The most important factor in the retention of a precision parallel dowel, as with any dowel, is length.[1-3, 5] Since no part of the dowel preparation developed by the standard Para-Post drill is rounded over or tapered, the dowel space tends to come closer to the exterior of the root at its apical extension. An assessment of the length of the dowel space should take this into account. The dowel should be at least as long as the clinical crown of the tooth,[6] or as long as possible without encroaching on the apical 4.0 mm. of the endodontic filling.

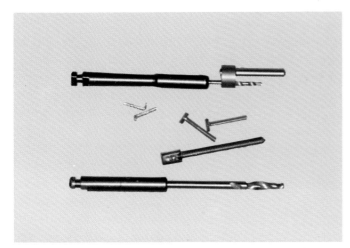

Fig. 7-1 The instruments and accessories needed for the fabrication of a direct Para-Post pattern are pictured here. Color coded plastic posts are available in diameters of 1.25 mm. (red), 1.50 mm. (black), and 1.75 mm. (green). Diameters of 0.9 mm. and 1.0 mm. can also be obtained. There is a paralleling jig for each of the diameters to be used in conjunction with a 0.7 mm. Paramax twist drill. Plastic pins are used for an impression if the indirect technique is employed, and iridioplatinum pins are used for the wax pattern and casting.

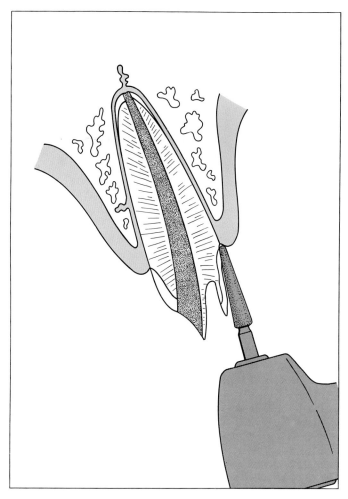

Fig. 7-2 A tooth being considered as a candidate for restoration with a Para-Post dowel-core should not be excessively tapered, and an adequate amount of tooth structure for pin placement should be present around the periphery of the canal.

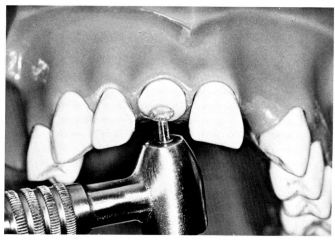

Fig. 7-3 All unsupported tooth structure is removed and the remaining root face is smoothed to provide a flat surface for pin placement.

165

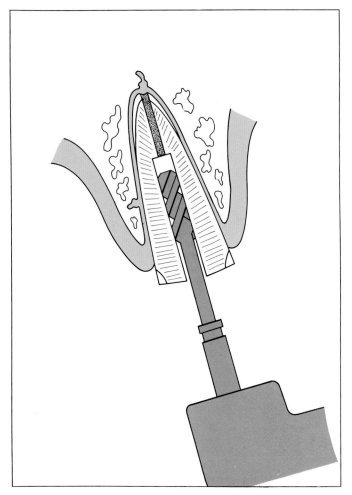

Fig. 7-4 The canal preparation is done, using the appropriate size of drill from the Para-Post kit. The dowel space should be at least as long as the clinical crown of the tooth to be restored, and longer if possible. Since the drill used is parallel-sided, the diameter of the root at the apical end of the dowel space is an important consideration. If the existing canal is too tapered, one should choose another technique for constructing the dowel-core.

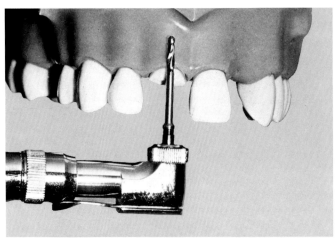

Fig. 7-5 The correct size of drill is shown superimposed over the facial of the tooth. The dowel space is instrumented with the selected drill after enlarging the canal initially with graduated sizes of Peeso reamers.

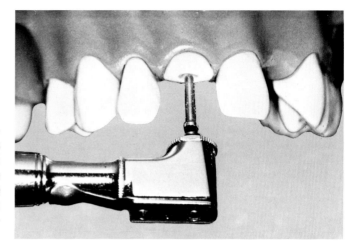

Fig. 7-6 Avoid excessive instrumentation, since this technique relies on the precision diameter of the dowel space to closely approximate that of the prefabricated dowel. Retention failures can result from over instrumentation with the drill.

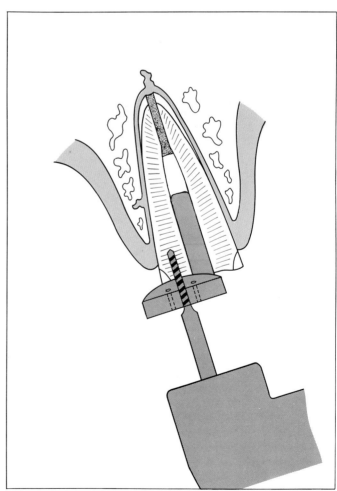

Fig. 7-7 The paralleling jig and a 0.7 mm. Paramax drill are used to place pin holes parallel with the dowel space.

167

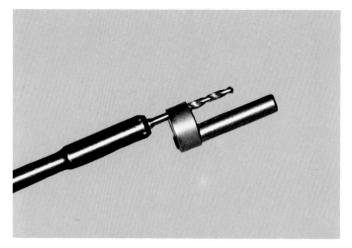

Fig. 7-8 The paralleling jig whose diameter corresponds with the drill used for the dowel preparation is selected. The length of the twist drill extending beyond the guide channel is adequate for instrumenting a deep pin hole.

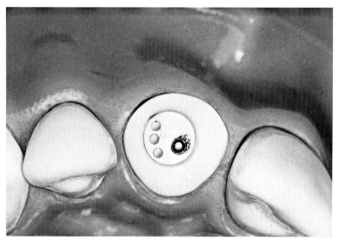

Fig. 7-9 The jig is placed in the prepared dowel space, and the guide channel that places the pin in the best position is selected. The guide channels are 0.5 mm., 0.8 mm., and 1.1 mm. away from the paralleling guide post. The guide channel chosen should place the pins in the area of the greatest bulk of tooth structure.

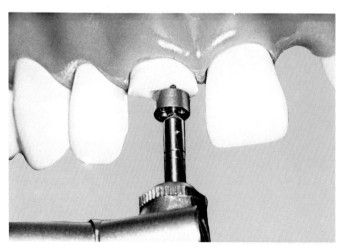

Fig. 7-10 The Paramax drill has a tapered shank which results in its being free-floating or unguided by the handpiece. Therefore, it can align itself with the selected channel, insuring that the pin hole will be parallel with the dowel preparation. The number of pins placed will be dictated by the available bulk of tooth structure. An attempt is made to place two pins. If possible, pin holes are drilled to the complete depth allowed by the paralleling jig.

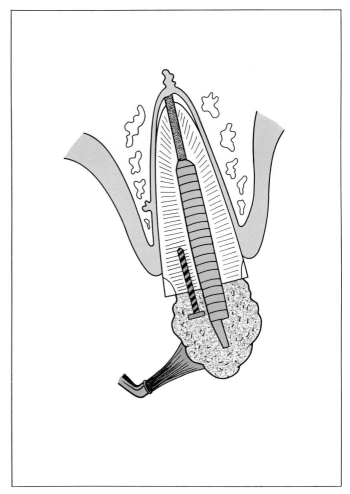

Fig. 7-11 After the plastic dowel pattern and iridioplatinum pins have been inserted, the core portion of the pattern is fabricated from autopolymerizing acrylic resin.*

* Duralay, Reliance Dental Mfg. Co., Chicago, IL.

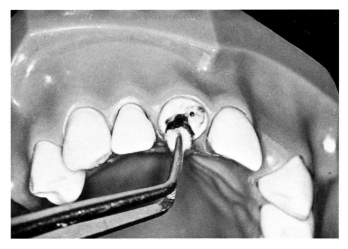

Fig. 7-12 The root face and any portion of the canal that may contact acrylic during core fabrication should be lubricated generously.

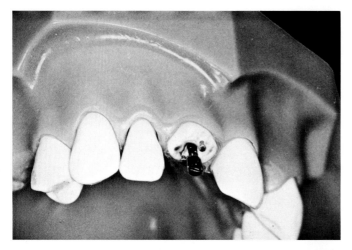

Fig. 7-13 The plastic dowel pattern and the iridioplatinum pins are now placed into their respective prepared spaces. Care should be taken to insure that the dowel is seated completely without fitting loosely.

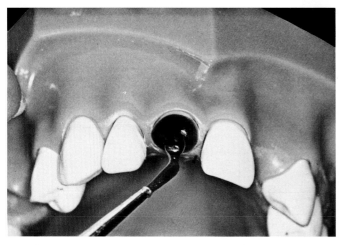

Fig. 7-14 A thin mix of Duralay acrylic is painted around the dowel and pins. If the dowel does not closely adapt in the coronal portion of the post space, or if any keyways have been prepared in the canal, resin is carefully placed into these areas.

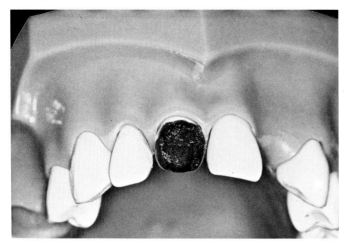

Fig. 7-15 The core is bulked up and allowed to polymerize. As the material becomes doughy, the pattern should be worked in and out of the tooth several times to insure that the pattern can be removed when completely set. If there are any voids or areas that need additional bulk, a second mix of resin can be added to the pattern.

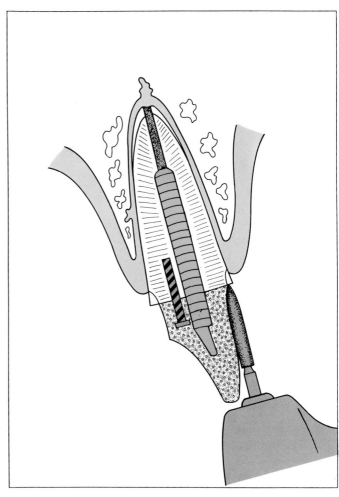

Fig. 7-16 Preparation of the core is accomplished, producing in it the contour of a crown preparation for a porcelain fused to metal crown.

Fig. 7-17 The gross reduction and most of the preparation of the core is completed out of the mouth. The pattern can be placed in the tooth occasionally to check for reduction and proper orientation of the preparation. Sandpaper discs and stones can be used for the contouring done in the hand. Finishing touches on the core preparation are accomplished on the tooth with a non-dentate tapered fissure bur.

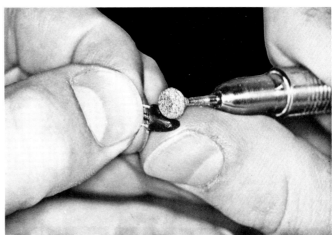

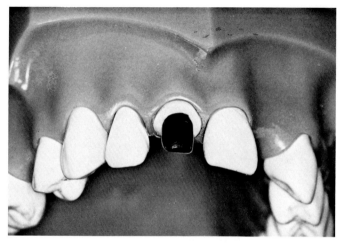

Fig. 7-18 The final preparation is evaluated for adequate reduction. Care is taken to insure that all finish lines for the final crown are on solid tooth structure, and not on the acrylic core. The preparation should be completed at this time, leaving little or nothing to be done when the dowel-core is in metal.

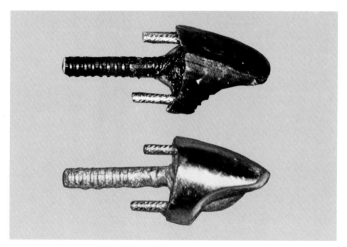

Fig. 7-19 The dowel-core pattern made with a Para-Post is seen top. The cast dowel-core after sprue removal and finishing is seen on the bottom. It is now ready to be tried in.

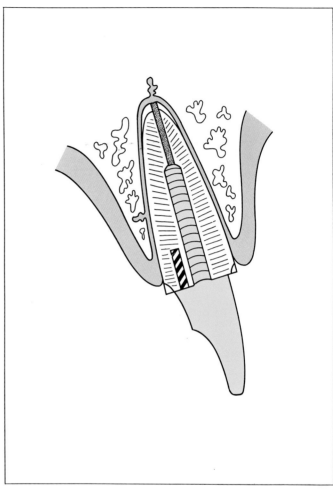

Fig. 7-20 The cast dowel-core is checked for complete seating and adequate fit. Any modifications needed on the core should be accomplished prior to cementation.

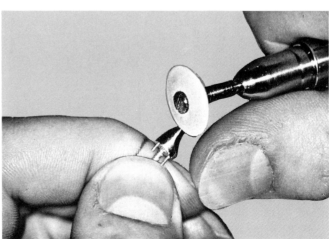

Fig. 7-21 After any changes are made in the dowel-core, the core portion is finished with a rubber wheel.

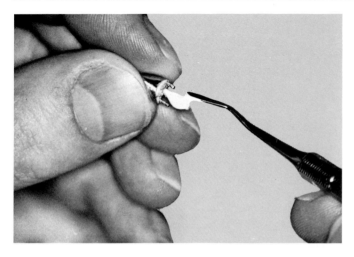

Fig. 7-22 The dowel is generously coated with a thin mix of
zinc phosphate cement.

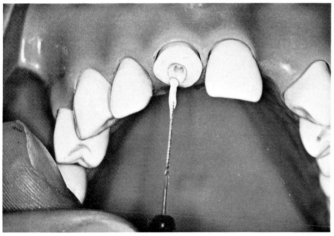

Fig. 7-23 Cement is applied to
the pin holes on a small endodontic file while the tooth is kept dry
and isolated.

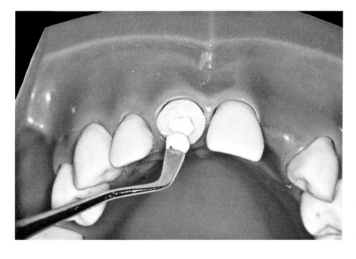

Fig. 7-24 Cement is placed in
the canal. If necessary, a Lentulo
spiral can be used to coat the
walls of the canal with cement.

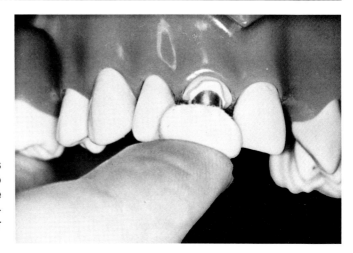

Fig. 7-25 The dowel-core is seated into the canal slowly to allow the cement to escape as the dowel goes to place. The restoration is held in place under finger pressure until the cement has set.

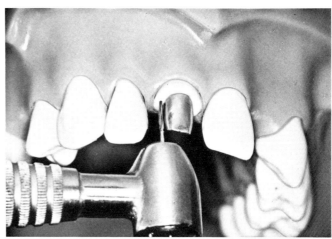

Fig. 7-26 The finish lines are extended to their final position, the junction between the core and tooth is smoothed, and any minor undercuts are removed.

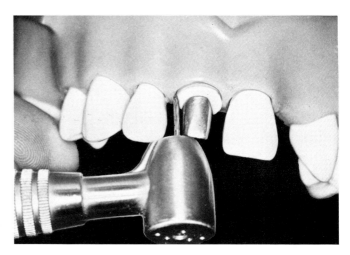

Fig. 7-27 A bevel is placed around the entire periphery of the preparation to complete it.

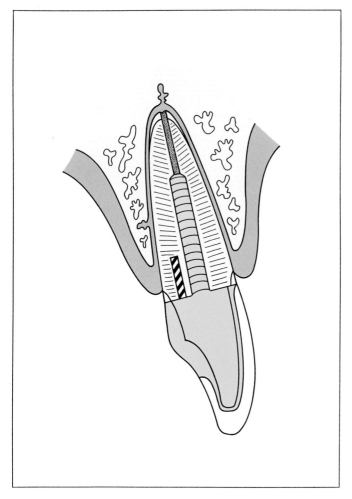

Fig. 7-28 The fabrication of the final crown is now accomplished. The dowel-core restoration is treated just as if it were a preparation in natural tooth structure.

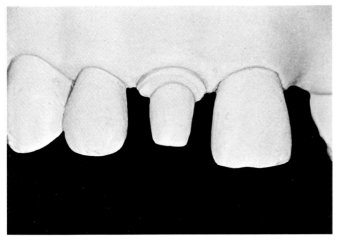

Fig. 7-29 When viewed on a stone cast, the preparation should appear to be an ideal one, except that no attempt has been made to conserve coronal tooth structure. Therefore, reduction in all dimensions should be more than adequate.

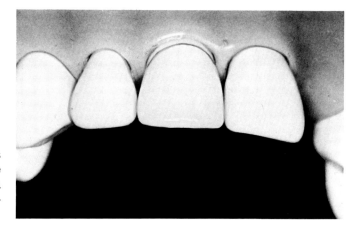

Fig. 7-30 The final crown is adjusted and cemented in the same manner as a crown on a preparation in natural tooth structure.

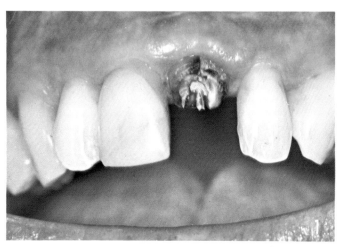

Fig. 7-31 This patient presented with a severely broken down maxillary central incisor. The previous endodontic obturation had been accomplished with a silver point. It was removed and replaced with a gutta percha filling at this time.

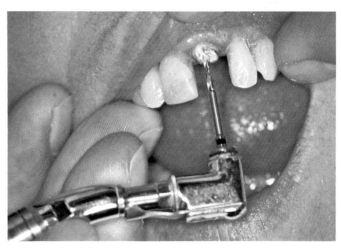

Fig. 7-32 The dowel space was prepared with a Para-Post drill.

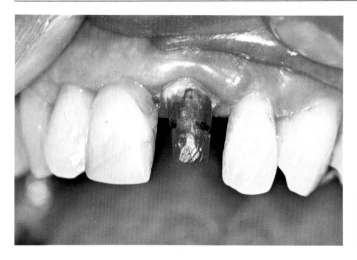

Fig. 7-33 The direct pattern was fabricated using the precision plastic dowel and Duralay resin to build up the core.

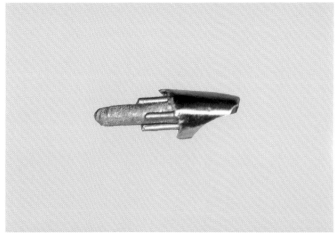

Fig. 7-34 The cast dowel-core has three parallel pins. Each pin hole was placed to the full length allowed by the paralleling jig and Paramax twist drill.

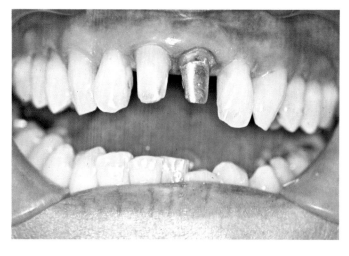

Fig. 7-35 The cemented dowel-core in the maxillary left central incisor and a porcelain fused to metal preparation in tooth structure on the maxillary right central incisor are ready for their final restorations.

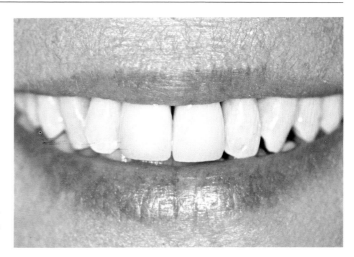

Fig. 7-36 The completed porcelain fused to metal crowns are seen after cementation.

References

1. Colley, I. T., Hampson, E. L. and Lehman, M. L.: Retention of post crowns: An assessment of the relative efficiency of posts of different shapes and sizes. *Brit Dent J,* 124:63–69, Jan. 1968.

2. Standlee, J. P., Caputo, A. A. and Hanson, E. C.: Retention of endodontic dowels: Effects of cement, dowel length, diameter, and design. *J Prosthet Dent,* 39:401–405, Apr. 1978.

3. Johnson, J. K. and Sakumura, J. S.: Dowel form and tensile force. *J Prosthet Dent,* 40:645–649, Dec. 1978.

4. Baraban, D. J.: A simplified method for making posts and cores. *J Prosthet Dent,* 24: 287–297, Sept. 1970.

5. Krupp, J. D., Caputo, A. A., Trabert, K. C. and Standlee, J. P.: Dowel retention with glass ionomer cement. *J Prosthet Dent,* 41:163–166, Feb. 1979.

6. McPherson, J. L.: A simplified root-dowel technique. *J So Calif St Dent Assoc,* 39:115–119, Feb. 1971.

Chapter 8

Precision Tapered Plastic Dowel

Most of the precision plastic dowel systems which are marketed today are tapered, with the taper ranging from 1.1° to 6.2°. Ideally, the use of a tapered precision plastic dowel with a matched reamer of the same size obviates the need for relining the dowel in the canal when the dowel-core is fabricated. The use of a taper is advocated by some authors because it more nearly approximates the tapered configuration of roots, thereby lessening the chance of a lateral perforation during dowel preparation.[1, 2] Tapered dowels exhibit the least stress during cementation, but they do tend to have a wedging effect.[3]

To match the tapered plastic pattern to the dowel preparation with accuracy, it may be necessary to cut a little length from the small end of the pattern, or reinstrument the canal to enlarge it slightly, depending on whether the dowel is too loose or too tight.[4] This must be done with great care, comparing the depth of the dowel preparation and the length of the dowel pattern. Otherwise, it is possible to wedge a tapered dowel into the canal, making contact with its walls short of full seating of the dowel.[5, 6] The operator may misinterpret the slight "tug back" that he feels as a manifestation of an accurate fit. The dowel can be relined,[7] of course, but that offsets much of the advantage of using a precision plastic dowel pattern.

The most commonly used precision plastic dowels will be described briefly. Although the technique will be given in detail for only that system which utilizes canal enlargement with hand instruments, the principles and general technique are essentially the same for all of them.

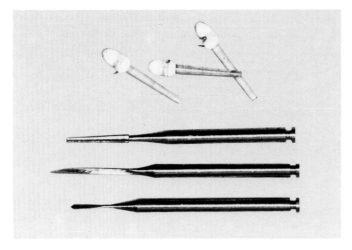

Fig. 8-1 The C · I (Calibrated Instrumentation) Kit* consists of three rotary instruments. The dowel preparation is begun with a bibevel twist drill. When the initial channel has been prepared, it is enlarged with a pointed reamer. The final diameter and taper is achieved with a tapered fissure bur whose size and taper match those of the dowel pattern. The smooth-sided patterns have a taper of 2.6°, and they are available in two sizes: 1.0–1.3 mm. and 1.2–1.6 mm. The two numbers in each set indicate the diameters at the tip and 10 mm. from the tip. There is a separate set of instruments for each dowel size.

* Parkell, Farmingdale, NY.

Fig. 8-2 There are five sizes of patterns in the Colorama Kit*: 0.8–1.3 mm., 0.9–1.4 mm., 1.0–1.6 mm., 1.0–1.8 mm., and 1.1–2.0 mm. The smooth sided dowel patterns are actually a combination of tapered and parallel-sided, with the tapered portion increasing in length from 5.0 mm. on the smallest dowel to 9.0 mm. on the largest. The tapered portion has a convergence angle of 6.2°. The dowel preparation is accomplished with a color-coded engine reamer of a matching size, which is tapered near the tip and parallel-sided adjacent to the shank.

* J. Aderer, Inc. (Metaux Precieux), Long Island City, NY.

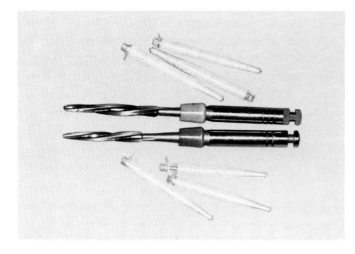

Fig. 8-3 P-D Posts* are smooth-sided plastic dowel patterns with a uniform convergence angle of 1.6°. The dowel space is prepared with a reamer of like taper and diameter. Each reamer has an adjustable sliding metal stop which is held in place with a set screw. The patterns are available in six sizes: 0.9–1.3 mm., 1.1–1.5 mm., 1.3–1.7 mm., 1.7–2.1 mm., and 1.9–2.3 mm.

* Union Broach Corp. (Produits Dentaires), Long Island City, NY.

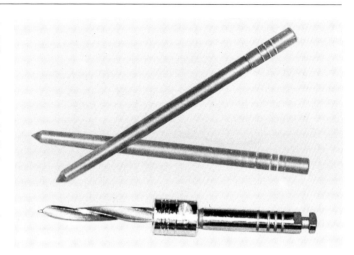

Fig. 8-4 The Endowel* system differs from the others in that its smooth tapered dowel patterns are matched to hand instruments, i.e., the standardized endodontic files and reamers. Therefore, they exhibit the 1.1° taper of standardized endodontic instruments. The dowels are available in eight sizes: 70 (0.7–0.9 mm.), 80 (0.8–1.0 mm.), 90 (0.9–1.1 mm.), 100 (1.0–1.2 mm.), 110 (1.1–1.3 mm.), 120 (1.2–1.4 mm.), 130 (1.3–1.5 mm.), and 140 (1.4–1.6 mm.). In each pair of numbers, the first designates diameter at the tip, while the second represents the diameter 10 mm. from the tip.

* Star Dental Mfg. Co., Inc., Conshohocken, PA.

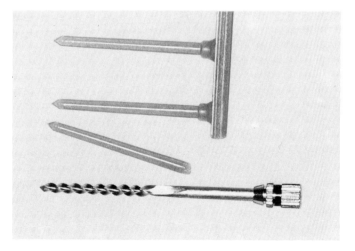

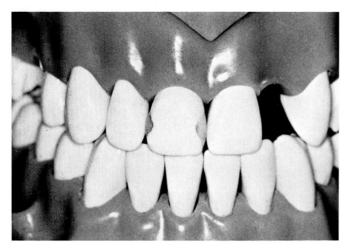

Fig. 8-5 The tapered dowel can be used in any of those situations requiring a dowel-core. They are especially useful in restoring teeth with moderately destroyed crowns which will have some coronal tooth structure remaining after the preparation has been completed.

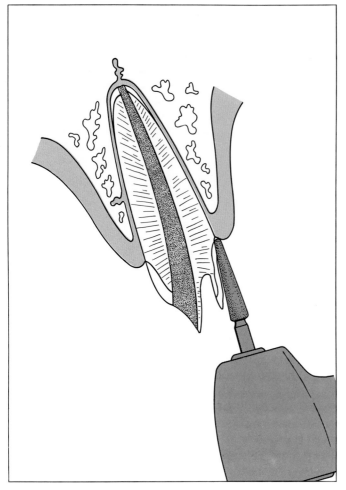

Fig. 8-6 The preparation for the dowel-core is begun by approximating the preparation for the final restoration, a porcelain fused to metal crown. This will facilitate fabrication of a properly contoured core pattern later.

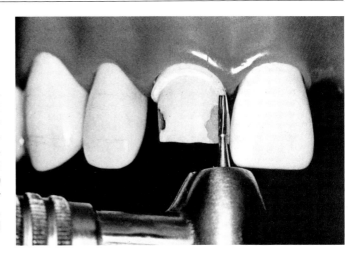

Fig. 8-7 The facial and proximal axial surfaces are planed with a No. 170 nondentate tapered fissure bur, after the axial reduction is done with a flat-end tapered diamond. The axial reduction is at least 1.25 mm. deep and incisal reduction should be 2.0 mm. A definite gingival shoulder is instrumented at this time. Caries, old restorations and bases will be dealt with later.

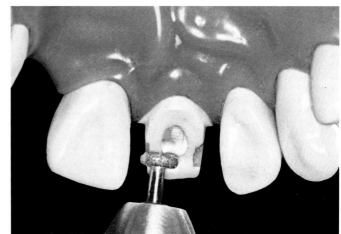

Fig. 8-8 Reduction of the lingual surface is begun by hollow grinding the cingulum to a depth of 1.0 mm. to produce a distinctly concave surface.

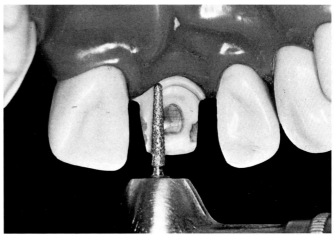

Fig. 8-9 If possible, a chamfer finish line is placed on the upright portion of the lingual surface with a round-end tapered diamond. When the cingulum wall is too short, a shoulder finish line is placed to move the lingual wall facially toward the center of the tooth. The bulk of tooth structure there should result in a longer lingual wall.

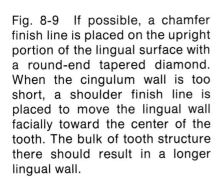

185

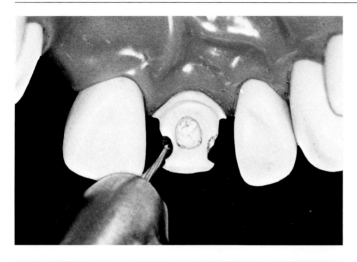

Fig. 8-10 Use a No. 4 or No. 6 round bur to excavate caries, bases, and any previous restorations.

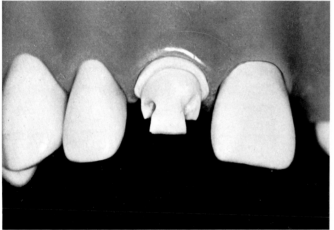

Fig. 8-11 The remaining tooth structure is evaluated to determine what can be retained and what must be removed. Since the presence of sound coronal tooth structure will increase dowel length without necessitating a deeper dowel preparation, as much tooth structure as possible should be preserved.

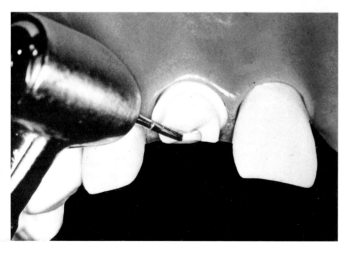

Fig. 8-12 A No. 170 nondentate tapered fissure bur is used to eliminate all unsupported and unusable tooth structure. As much supragingival coronal tooth structure as possible is preserved.

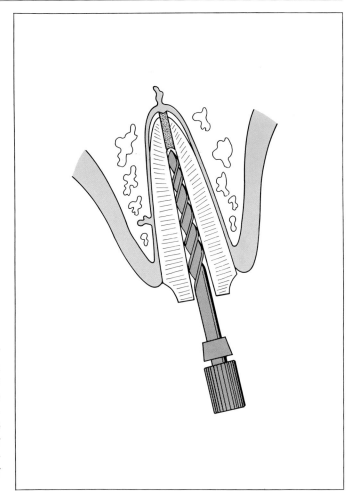

Fig. 8-13 The tooth is ready for preparation of the dowel space. A series of hand files will be used to enlarge and lengthen the canal to the desired size. Because standardized endodontic hand files are used, this step could be nearly completed at the time of endodontic treatment and merely touched up at this point.

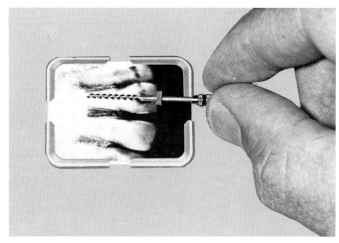

Fig. 8-14 The file is measured against a radiograph of the tooth being restored. Place a rubber stop on the file to serve as an indicator of preparation depth. The dowel should be two-thirds the length of the canal and should stop at least 4.0 mm. short of the apex.

187

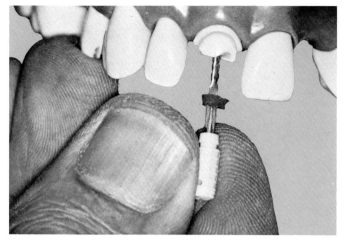

Fig. 8-15 After removing as much gutta percha as possible with a hot endodontic plugger, start the canal preparation with the largest file that will fit into the canal. Smaller diameter Peeso reamers can be used for the initial instrumentation. Make another radiograph to verify the accuracy of preparation depth.

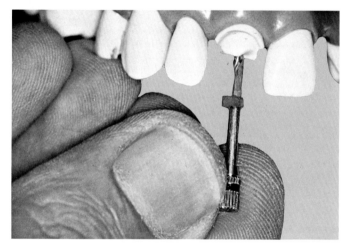

Fig. 8-16 Continue enlarging the canal until the desired diameter and length have been achieved. Do not over instrument the canal, or the advantage of a precision pattern will be lost and the dowel will require relining.

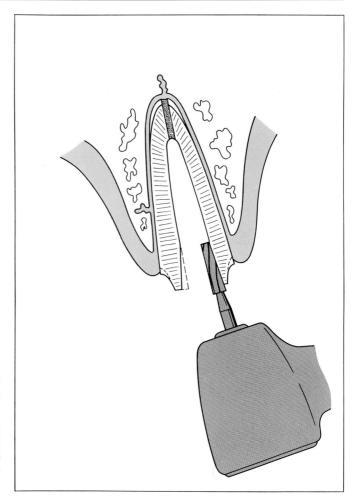

Fig. 8-17 A keyway should be placed at the mouth of the canal to provide anti-rotational resistance. Vertical grooves 3–4 mm. long are used on single rooted teeth, and a short dowel in a second canal is used on multi-rooted teeth.

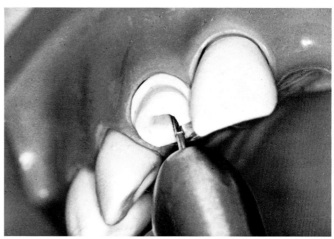

Fig. 8-18 Make the keyway 1.0 mm. deep, which is the diameter of the No. 170 bur used for placing it. It should be located in the area of greatest bulk. A contrabevel is added around the entire occlusal external periphery of the preparation.

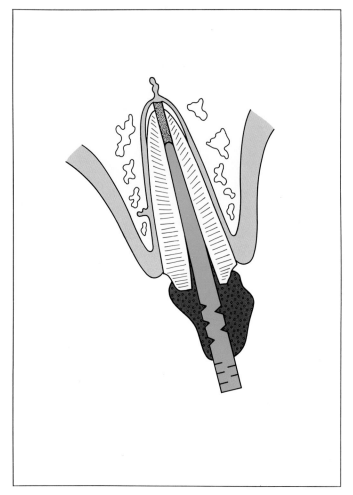

Fig. 8-19 The dowel-core pattern will be fabricated with the corresponding size of tapered plastic Endowel pattern. It can be used for making an impression for the indirect technique, or a direct core can be attached to the dowel in the tooth. Both wax[4, 8] and resin[4] have been described for this purpose.

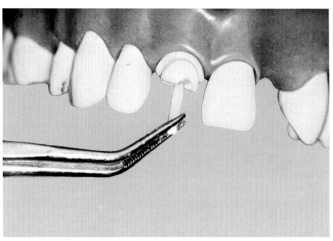

Fig. 8-20 Try the appropriate size of plastic dowel in the canal. It should fit into the canal without resistance and without flopping from side to side. To insure complete seating, compare the length of the pattern with the depth of the preparation, using a periodontal probe or a smaller diameter dowel pattern.

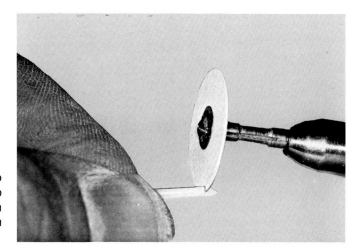

Fig. 8-21 If the dowel fits too loosely, use a sandpaper disc to remove 1 mm. increments from the apical end until it fits closely in the canal.

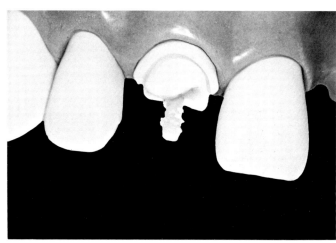

Fig. 8-22 If the plastic dowel fits well, excess occlusal length is removed from the coronal end of the dowel pattern. Roughen 2 or 3 mm. to aid retention of the resin core.

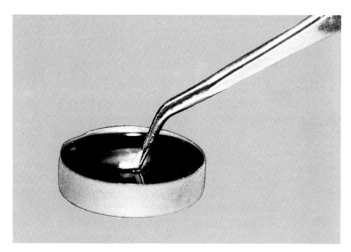

Fig. 8-23 Use a cotton pellet to transfer lubricant to the dowel preparation.

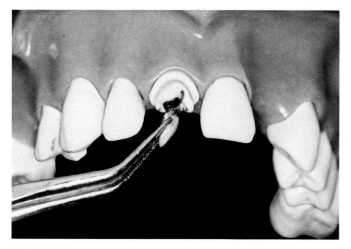

Fig. 8-24 Apply the lubricant liberally to the root face and the orifice of the canal. Since the dowel will not be relined, it is not necessary to get lubricant all the way to the end of the dowel preparation.

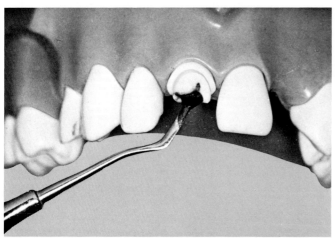

Fig. 8-25 Mix resin* to a runny consistency and place a small amount in the mouth of the canal, making sure that it extends into the keyways.

* Duralay, Reliance Dental Mfg. Co., Chicago, IL.

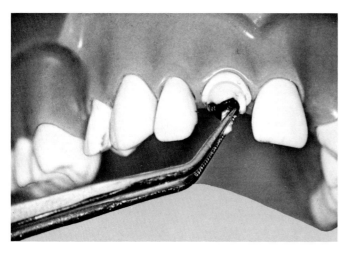

Fig. 8-26 Place the tapered dowel pattern into the canal until it touches the apical end of the dowel preparation. All of the external contrabevel should be covered with resin at this time.

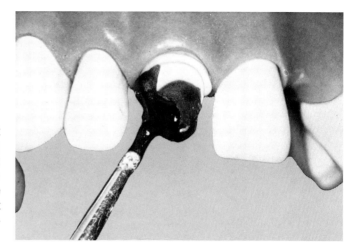

Fig. 8-27 Add resin around that portion of the dowel protruding from the canal to provide the bulk needed for a core. When the resin becomes doughy, pump the dowel in and out to prevent it from becoming locked into undercuts in the canal.

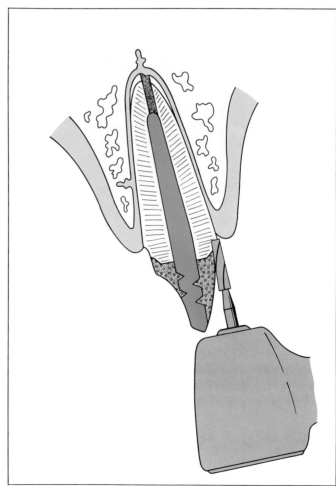

Fig. 8-28 Shape the coronal bulk of resin to form it into a crown preparation for the restoration which will ultimately be placed on the tooth.

193

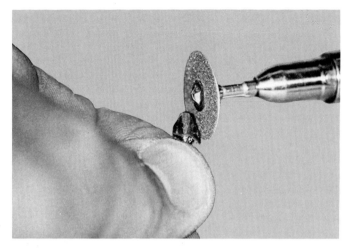

Fig. 8-29 The pattern is removed from the tooth so the axial surfaces can be formed with a coarse garnet disc. Replace the pattern in the canal occasionally to keep the contours of the core consistent with those of the remaining coronal tooth structure.

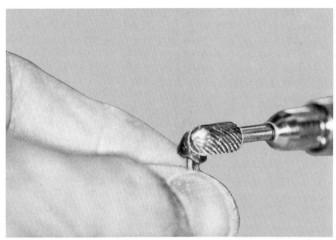

Fig. 8-30 Shape the concave lingual surface with a large acrylic bur.

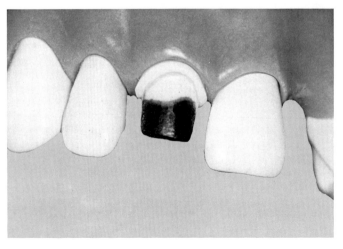

Fig. 8-31 Replace the pattern in the tooth for the finishing touches. The axial surfaces can be smoothed on the tooth with a nondentate tapered fissure bur. This important step should be completed in acrylic because it is time-consuming to shape the dowel-core after it has been cast in nickel-chrome.

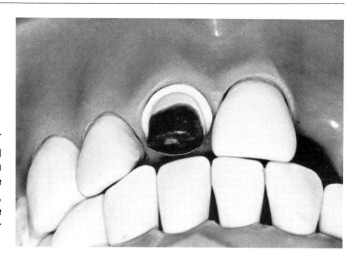

Fig. 8-32 Check the pattern for clearance with the opposing teeth. Is there space for a crown between the pattern and the opposing incisal edges? If not, more reduction should be done now. Plastic is decidedly softer than nickel-chrome.

Fig. 8-33 Attach the sprue to the incisal edge with sticky wax and place the sprue in the crucible former. Use a carbon-free high-heat phosphate-bonded investment* for a nickel-chrome dowel-core and a gypsum-bonded investment** for a gold alloy dowel-core.

 * High Temp Investment, Whip-Mix Corporation, Louisville, KY.
** Beauty Cast Investment, Whip-Mix Corporation, Louisville, KY.

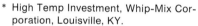

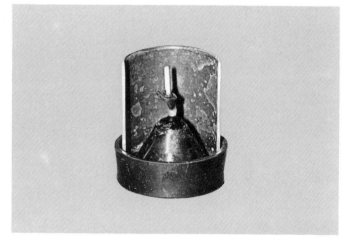

Fig. 8-34 The dowel-core pattern, using a precision tapered dowel, is shown above with the cast dowel-core below it.

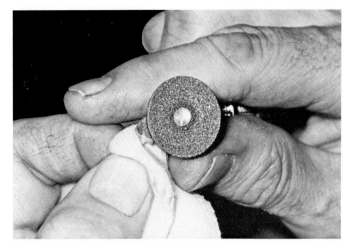

Fig. 8-35 Remove the sprue with a 7/8 inch Carborundum disc or a 1½ inch cut-off disc. Rough trimming, especially around the sprue attachment, is done with the Carborundum disc. Finish contouring the surfaces around the sprue with a No. 8 aluminum oxide pink wheel on a mandrel.

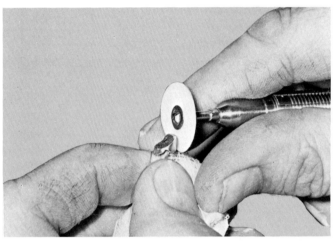

Fig. 8-36 A matte surface can be achieved on the core portion by smoothing it first with coarse garnet disks and then with finer sandpaper discs.

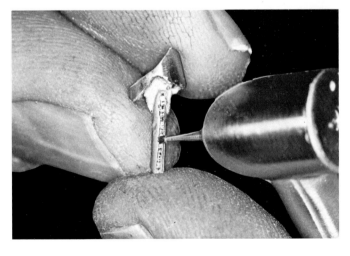

Fig. 8-37 Use a No. 35 or 56 carbide bur to place the cement vent on the side of the dowel. This task can be simplified on nickel-chrome dowel-cores if the groove is cut first in the plastic dowel pattern and then retouched in the finished casting.

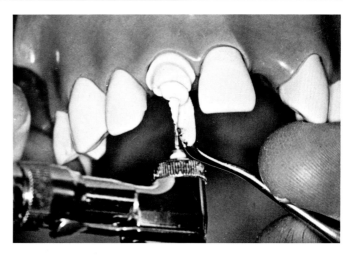

Fig. 8-38 Insert a portion of a thin mix of zinc phosphate cement into the mouth of the dried and isolated canal. Hold a plastic instrument dripping with cement immediately adjacent to the canal and insert a slowly rotating Lentulo spiral through the fluid cement. In a few seconds, the spiral will carry the cement into the canal and coat the walls of the dowel space.

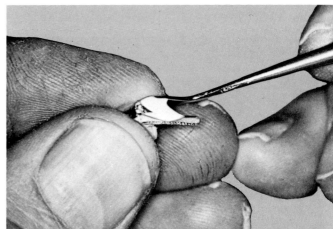

Fig. 8-39 Cover the dowel completely with the liquid cement and then insert the dowel slowly into the canal.

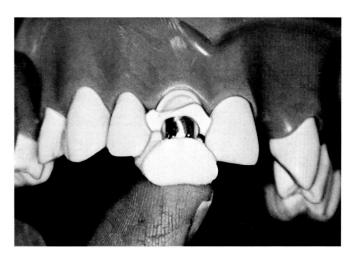

Fig. 8-40 Complete the seating of the dowel with finger pressure on a cotton roll. Do it slowly enough to allow the cement to escape ahead of the dowel.

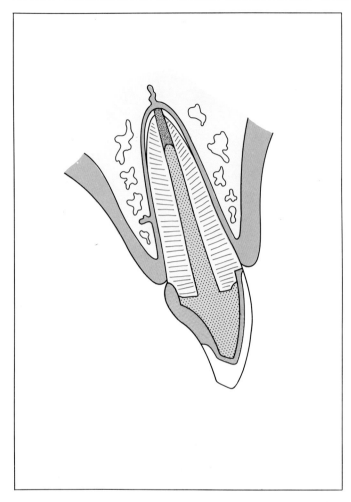

Fig. 8-41 The tooth is ready to be restored with a crown, treating that portion of coronal tooth form which has been built up with the core as though it were tooth structure.

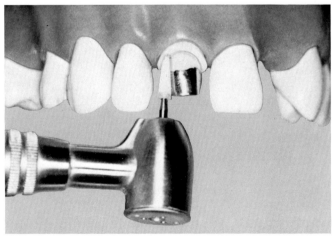

Fig. 8-42 A white polishing stone is used on the axial surfaces of the core and tooth to remove minor undercuts near the margin of the dowel-core.

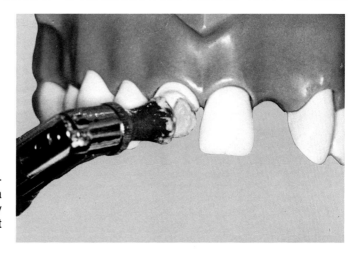

Fig. 8-43 Finish the axial surfaces of the core with pumice in a rubber cup. This will remove any remaining particles of cement while leaving a matte surface.

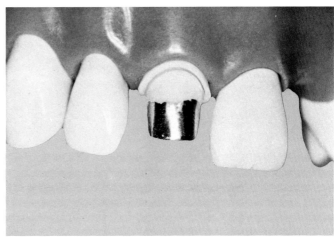

Fig. 8-44 Labial view of the completed dowel-core fabricated from a precision plastic dowel pattern.

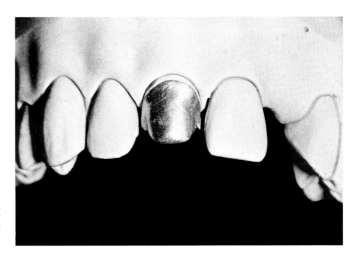

Fig. 8-45 The coping and porcelain fused to metal restoration are fabricated on a die and cast made from an impression of the tooth with the dowel-core.

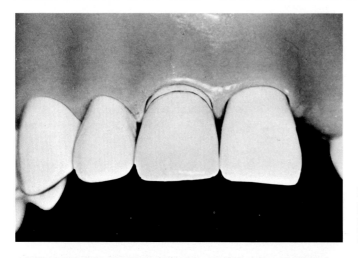

Fig. 8-46 The final restoration, a porcelain fused to metal crown, is placed over the tooth which has been built up with a dowel-core.

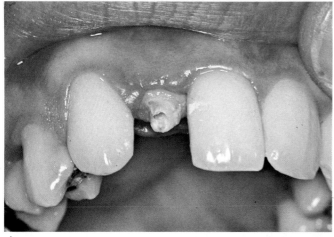

Fig. 8-47 This lateral incisor had no coronal tooth structure remaining after undermined segments of the crown had been removed.

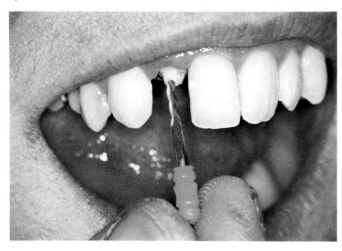

Fig. 8-48 The canal was instrumented to a No. 140 endodontic file.

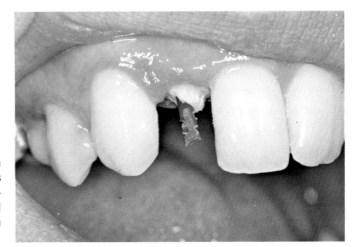

Fig. 8-49 A No. 140 precision plastic Endowel pattern was placed in the canal. It was shortened at the incisal end and roughened to improve retention of the resin core.

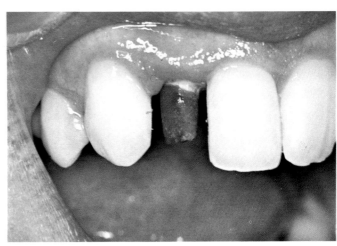

Fig. 8-50 The core was built up with resin and trimmed to form a porcelain fused to metal crown preparation.

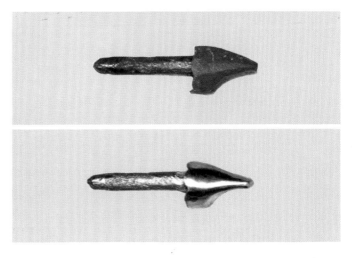

Fig. 8-51 The completed dowel-core pattern is seen before investing (top). After burnout, and casting, it was finished for cementation (bottom).

201

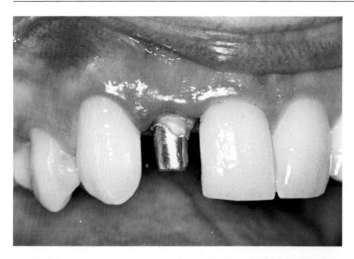

Fig. 8-52 The completed En-dowel dowel-core is seen after cementation, ready for fabrica-tion of the final restoration.

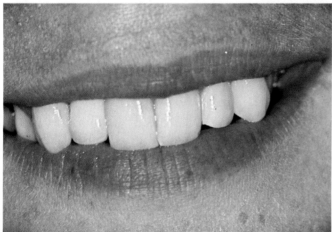

Fig. 8-53 The porcelain fused to metal crown provided an esthetic and functional restoration of the tooth that would not have been possible without building up the tooth first.

References

1. Johnson, J. K., Schwartz, N. L. and Blackwell, R. T.: Evaluation and restoration of endodontically treated posterior teeth. *JADA,* 93:597–605, Sept. 1976.

2. Miller, A. W.: Direct pattern technique for posts and cores. *J Prosthet Dent,* 40:392–397, Oct. 1978.

3. Standlee, J. P., Caputo, A. A., Collard, E. W. and Pollack, M. H.: Analysis of stress distribution of endodontic posts. *Oral Surg,* 33:952–960, Jun. 1972.

4. Weine, F. S., Kahn, H., Wax, A. H. and Taylor, G. N.: The use of standardized tapered plastic pins in post and core fabrication. *J Prosthet Dent,* 29:542–548, May 1973.

5. Baum, L.: Dowel placements in the endodontically treated tooth. *J Conn St Dent Assoc,* 53:116–117, Summer 1979.

6. Lau, V. S. M.: The reinforcement of endodontically treated teeth. *Dent Clin N Amer,* 20:313–328, Apr. 1976.

7. Jacoby, W. E.: Practical technique for the fabrication of a direct pattern for a post-core restoration. *J Prosthet Dent,* 35:357–360, Mar. 1976.

8. Kahn, H., Fishman, I. and Malone, W. F.: A simplified method for constructing a core following endodontic treatment. *J Prosthet Dent,* 37:32–36, Jan. 1977.

Chapter 9

Prefabricated Dowel/Cast Core

Another approach to the fabrication of dowel-cores has been one in which a precision made prefabricated dowel is matched in size to a bur or hand reamer. After the dowel preparation is completed, the prefabricated dowel is fit in the canal. A core is then made of resin or wax by either the direct or indirect technique. The metal dowel and its attached core pattern are invested, and the core is burned out. Then the core is cast in metal.

The principle employed is still one of making the canal fit the dowel rather than making the dowel fit the canal. The use of a prefabricated dowel with a cast core offers the advantage of having part of the dowel-core already completed before the procedure is even begun. It has also been promoted because of the superior strength of a wrought or drawn dowel compared with a cast one,[1-4] especially when the dowel is less than 1.5 mm. in diameter.[5]

The prefabricated dowels have been made of a variety of materials: gold,[6] gold-platinum-palladium,[7] iridioplatinum,[6] platinized wire,[8] nickel-cobalt-chromium,[5] and stainless steel.[2] In one technique, the dowel is used with a silver sleeve which is inserted in the canal before the dowel.[6] The core can be fabricated by the direct[6, 7, 9] or the indirect technique.[3, 4, 8, 10, 11]

Both parallel and tapered dowels have been made for this technique. A commonly used system has been the Endo-Post*, which utilizes a noble metal smooth tapered dowel which is matched to the standardized endodontic hand files and reamers.[3, 4, 9-11] A serrated, parallel-sided noble metal dowel used with a matching size twist drill is also available.**

* Endo-Post, Kerr Dental Mfg. Co., Romulus, MI.
** Para-Post, Whaledent International, New York, NY.

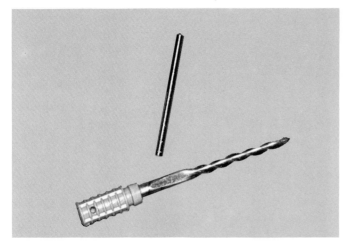

Fig. 9-1 The Endo-Post system utilizes a noble metal dowel which exhibits the slight 1.1° taper of the standardized endodontic instruments. It is available in eight sizes which match the size of endodontic files: 70 (0.7–0.9 mm.), 80 (0.8–1.0 mm.), 90 (0.9–1.1 mm.), 100 (1.0–1.2 mm.), 110 (1.1–1.3 mm.), 120 (1.2–1.4 mm.), 130 (1.3–1.5 mm.), and 140 (1.4–1.6 mm.).

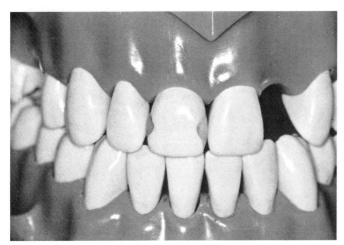

Fig. 9-2 A prefabricated dowel can be used in the fabrication of any dowel-core. Its use does not require that all remaining coronal tooth structure be destroyed.

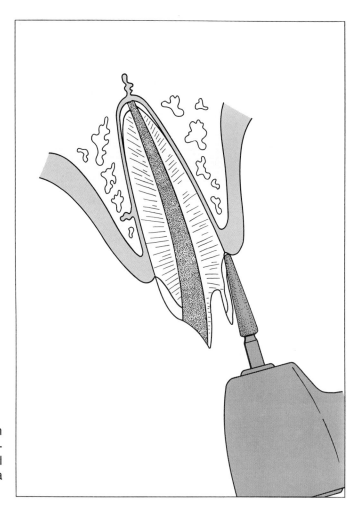

Fig. 9-3 Begin the preparation of the tooth for this type of dowel-core by producing the coronal contours of a preparation for a porcelain fused to metal crown.

Fig. 9-4 Axial reduction is accomplished with a flat-end tapered diamond. Then it is planed smooth with a No. 170 nondentate tapered fissure bur, instrumenting a definite gingival shoulder at the same time. There must be a minimum of 1.25 mm. reduction on the axial surfaces and 2.0 mm. on the incisal.

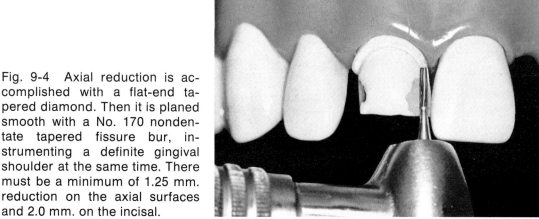

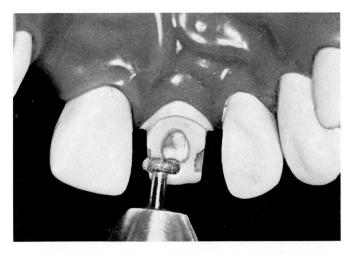

Fig. 9-5 The first step in the reduction of the lingual surface is the hollow grinding of the cingulum to a depth of 1.0 mm. The result should be a definite concavity over the entire cingulum surface.

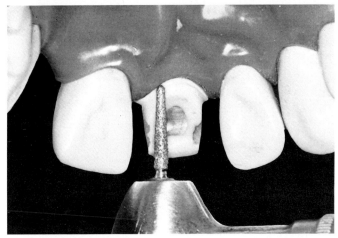

Fig. 9-6 With a round-end tapered diamond, produce an upright lingual wall to oppose the facial surface and give the preparation maximum retention. Ideally, a chamfer is desired for the linguo-gingival finish line. However, it may be necessary to use a shoulder if the cingulum is so short that the lingual wall will have no length otherwise.

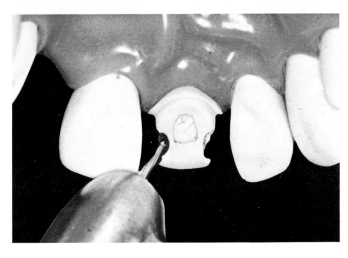

Fig. 9-7 Remove all caries, bases, and previous restorations with a round bur.

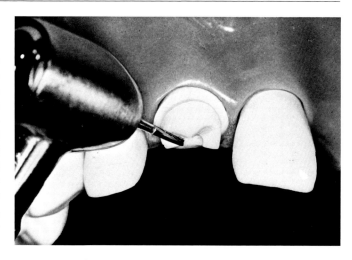

Fig. 9-8 Remaining tooth structure should be examined carefully and evaluated. Weak, undermined tooth structure which could break off later and compromise the strength of the restored tooth is removed now with a No. 170 bur. Wholesale destruction of all coronal tooth structure, sound as well as weakened, is to be avoided, however. It unnecessarily shortens the dowel.

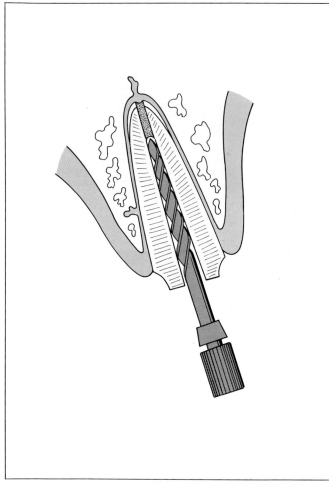

Fig. 9-9 The tooth is ready for preparation of the canal with a series of standardized hand files to produce the desired dowel length and diameter.

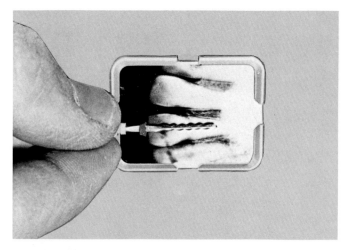

Fig. 9-10 Measure the file on a radiograph of the tooth being restored. Place a rubber stop on the instrument to indicate maximum penetration of the file. Make the dowel preparation at least as long as the crown length and stop 4.0 mm. short of the apical end of the root canal filling.

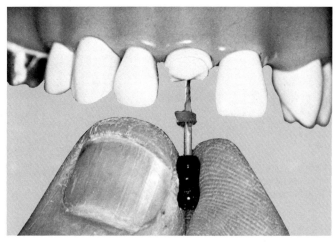

Fig. 9-11 Remove as much gutta percha as possible with a hot endodontic plugger before inserting the file which is next in the series after the last one used. When the file has been used to instrument the canal to the desired depth, make a radiograph to verify the accuracy of preparation length.

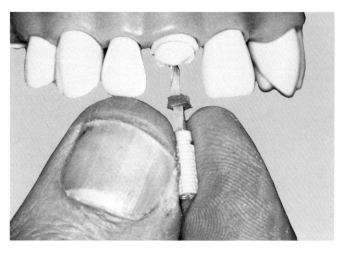

Fig. 9-12 Continue the enlargement of the canal until it is the desired length and diameter. Guard against over instrumenting the canal or a loose, sloppy fit will result. This type of dowel cannot be relined.

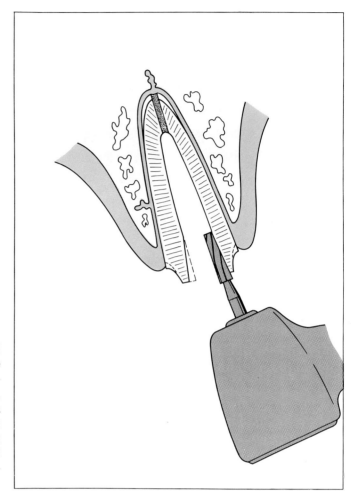

Fig. 9-13 An anti-rotational feature must be added to the canal. Vertical grooves are usually used on single-rooted teeth, while short auxillary dowels in a second canal are employed in multi-rooted teeth. Accessory pin holes have also been described for that purpose with the Endo-Post.[9]

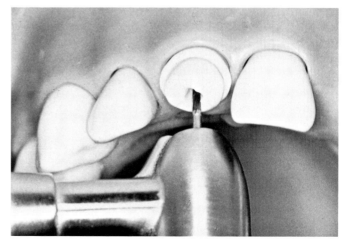

Fig. 9-14 Prepare the keyway to the length of the cutting flutes of the bur and sink it into the bulkiest wall of the canal to the diameter of the bur at the mouth of the canal. It should fade out at its apical end.

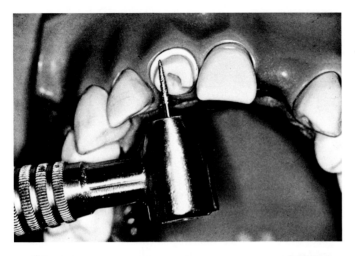

Fig. 9-15 Place a contra bevel around the entire external occlusal periphery of the dowel-core preparation, using a fine grit flame diamond or a No. 170 bur.

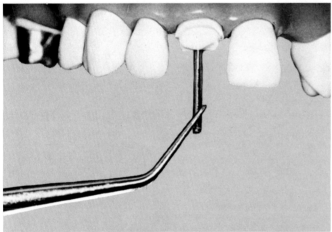

Fig. 9-16 Try the appropriate size of prefabricated dowel in the canal. It should fit the canal both without binding and without falling from side-to-side. To check on the seating of the dowel, compare its seated depth with that of a smaller dowel or a periodontal probe.

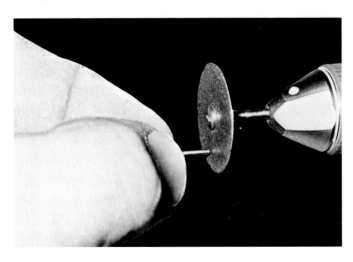

Fig. 9-17 If the dowel is loose in the canal, use a Carborundum separating disc to remove 1.0 mm. increments from the apical end of the dowel until it fits properly in the canal.

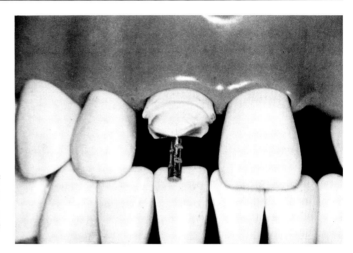

Fig. 9-18 Once the proper fit of the prefabricated metal dowel has been established in the canal, check its length by having the patient close his teeth together.

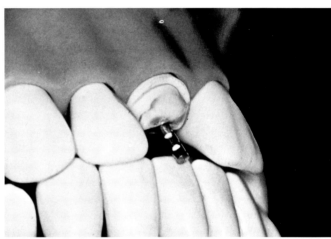

Fig. 9-19 Check the clearance of the dowel with teeth in the opposing arch.

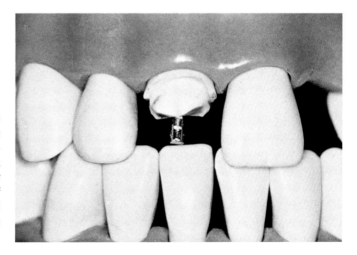

Fig. 9-20 If it is necessary to shorten the dowel, do it from the incisal end with the same Carborundum separating disc in a low speed handpiece. Grind a few shallow notches in the sides of the incisal segment of the dowel to enhance mechanical retention of the core.

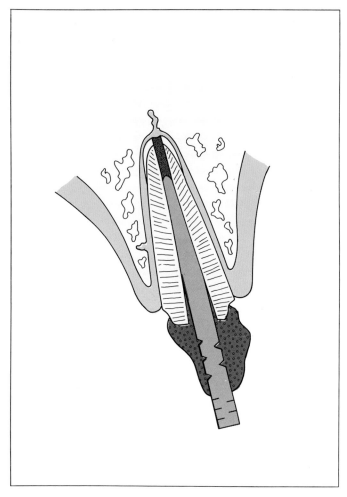

Fig. 9-21 A resin* core is fabricated around the incisal end of the prefabricated dowel which extends from the tooth. The dowel can also be used for making an impression of the dowel in order to fabricate the core indirectly.

* Duralay, Reliance Dental Mfg., Co., Chicago, IL.

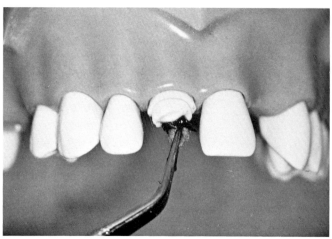

Fig. 9-22 Use a cotton pellet to apply lubricant to the face of the root and the canal orifice. It is not necessary to force lubricant all the way to the apical area of the dowel preparation, since the dowel is already completed.

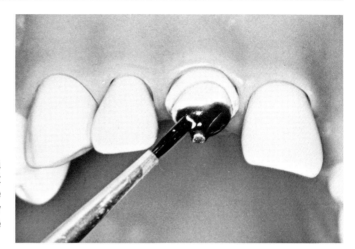

Fig. 9-23 Mix the resin to a runny consistency and apply it around the dowel in the canal. Be sure that it is placed in the keyway and any irregularities around the mouth of the canal.

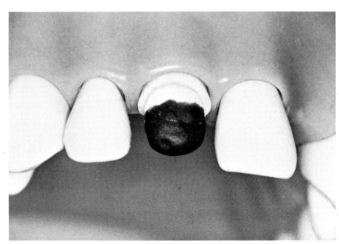

Fig. 9-24 Build up a large enough bulk of acrylic resin to provide a core that will have both the bulk and the contours of an ideal crown preparation for a porcelain fused to metal crown preparation.

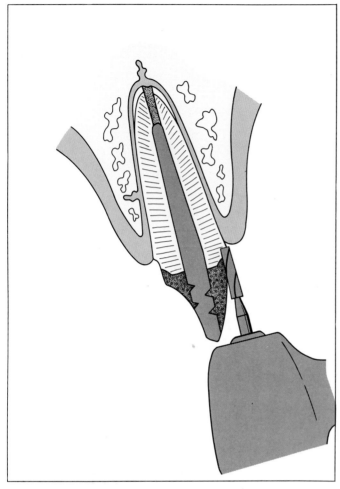

Fig. 9-25 The resin will be formed into the shape of a crown preparation for the final restoration.

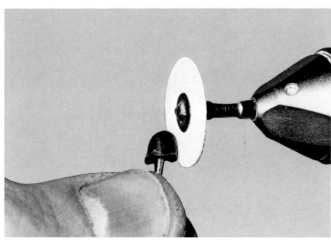

Fig. 9-26 Remove the pattern from the tooth and shape the axial surface with a coarse garnet disc. Finish the axial surfaces with a fine sandpaper disc.

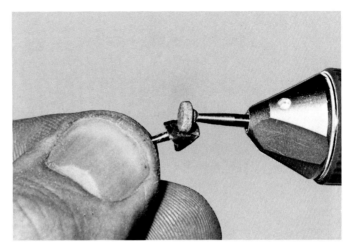

Fig. 9-27 Use a small Carborundum wheel to produce a concave surface on the lingual aspect of the core.

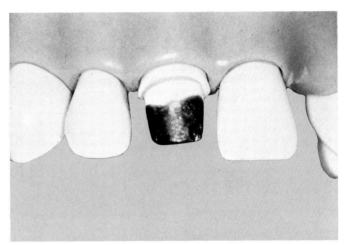

Fig. 9-28 Return the pattern to the tooth to insure that the contours of the core are consistent with those of the remaining coronal tooth structure. Finishing touches can be applied with a nondentate tapered fissure bur. Small voids or miscontoured areas can be corrected by brushing on alternating layers of monomer and polymer and then reshaping them. It is difficult or impossible to make these changes once the dowel-core has been cast.

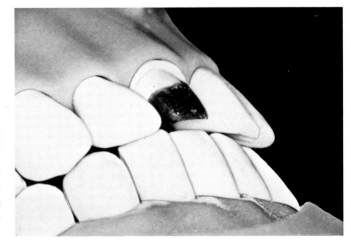

Fig. 9-29 Observe the pattern in place for clearance with opposing teeth. There must be space between the lingual surface of the pattern and the opposing incisal edges for a crown. If the space does not exist, it should be created now.

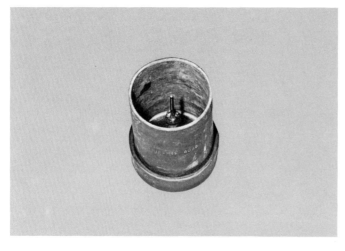

Fig. 9-30   Attach the sprue to the greatest bulk of the resin core pattern to insure that the casting alloy will completely surround the head of the prefabricated dowel. Invest the pattern in a gypsum-bonded investment.* To insure a good mechanical bond between dowel and cast core, a gold alloy should be used for the core.

* Beauty-Cast Investment, Whip-Mix Corporation, Louisville, KY.

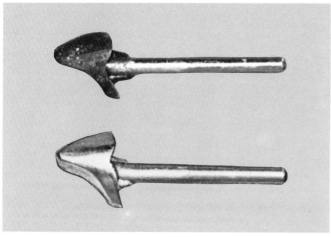

Fig. 9-31   The resin core completely surrounds the dowel, with the keyways extending down the dowel (top). The completed dowel-core with cast core is seen (bottom).

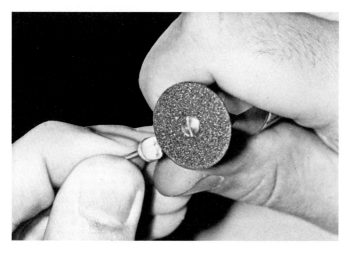

Fig. 9-32   The sprue is cut off with a 7/8 inch Carborundum separating disc. The area around the sprue attachment is trimmed with the same disc. A coarse rubber wheel can then be used on the entire core to smooth out uneven areas.

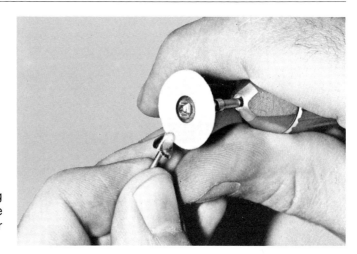

Fig. 9-33   Complete the finishing process by going over all of the core surface with a sandpaper disc.

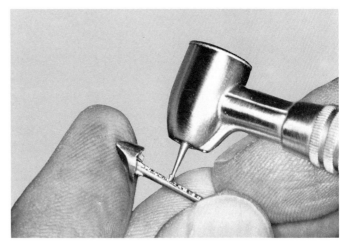

Fig. 9-34   Use a No. 35 carbide bur to place the v-shaped cement vent along the length of the dowel.

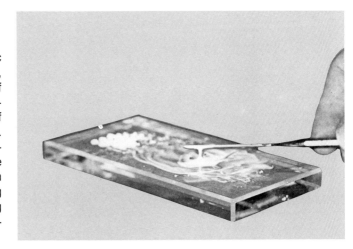

Fig. 9-35   A thin mix of zinc phosphate cement is made, spreading it over a wide area of the glass mixing slab and incorporating small increments of powder as the mix progresses. This is important to the successful completion of the dowel-core because properly mixed thin cement permits complete seating of the dowel without exerting undue lateral stress in the process.

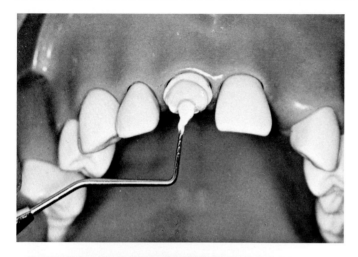

Fig. 9-36 The cement is placed in the canal with a Lentulo spiral or by use of a periodontal probe or thin endodontic plugger. The walls of the canal should be covered thoroughly with cement.

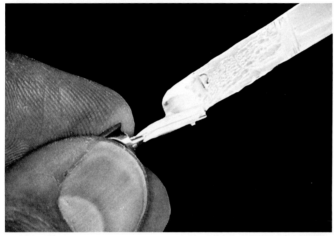

Fig. 9-37 Completely coat the dowel with cement.

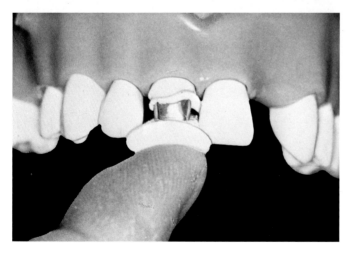

Fig. 9-38 Seat the dowel-core by using finger pressure over a cotton roll. Release the pressure every few seconds as the dowel is being inserted to allow back pressure to release itself along the vent. Reapply pressure to overcome rebound, and continue seating the dowel-core until it is in completely. Then hold finger pressure on it for about two minutes.

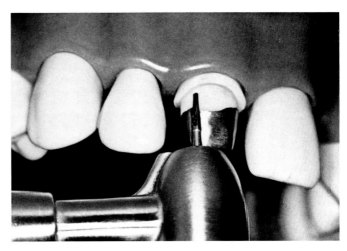

Fig. 9-39 Use a rotary instrument, such as a nondentate tapered fissure bur, to smooth the axial surfaces in proximity to the margins of the core. There should be no change in contour or depressions in the axial surfaces. These would produce problem causing undercuts when the porcelain fused to metal crown is fabricated.

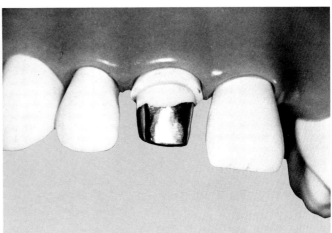

Fig. 9-40 The central incisor has been built up to the contours of an ideal tooth preparation for a porcelain fused to metal crown.

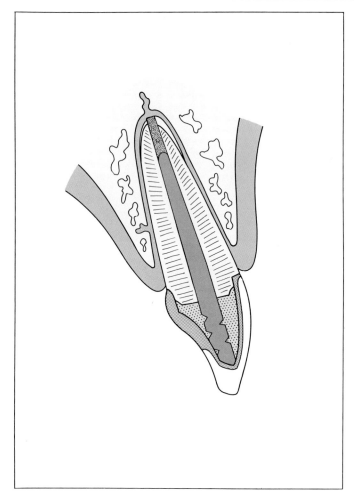

Fig. 9-41 The final restoration can be placed over the Endo-Post dowel-core as though it were virgin tooth structure.

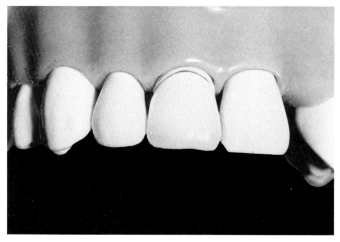

Fig. 9-42 The completed porcelain fused to metal restoration is shown in place over the dowelcore.

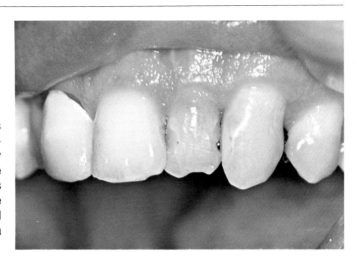

Fig. 9-43 This lateral incisor is riddled with interconnecting restorations and weakened by traumatically induced fracture lines. A full veneer crown was required to restore it, and there was not enough sound coronal tooth structure to support a crown.

Fig. 9-44 After removal of the unsupported tooth structure on this small tooth, there was virtually no remaining coronal tooth structure. The canal was instrumented to the size of a No. 130 file.

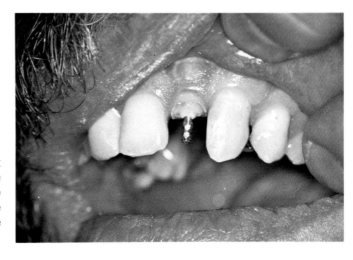

Fig. 9-45 A No. 130 Endo-Post was fitted, leaving 3.0 mm. of the incisal end protruding from the canal. Sides of the dowel were roughened to aid retention of the core.

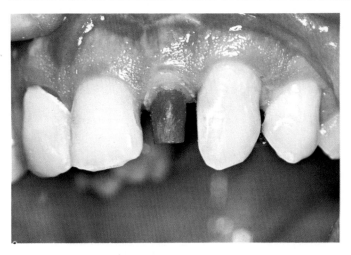

Fig. 9-46 A resin core was fabricated around the dowel.

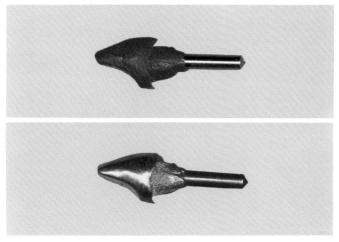

Fig. 9-47 The dowel with resin core is seen above, and the cast Endo-Post dowel-core is seen below. The core extends 2–3 mm. down the dowel providing a better union between dowel and core. This was done because of flaring of the incisal 20% of the dowel preparation.

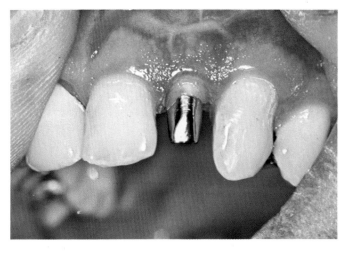

Fig. 9-48 The completed Endo-Post dowel-core is seen after its cementation. The tooth is now ready for its final restoration.

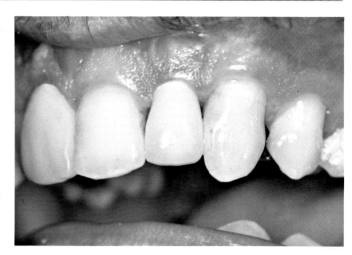

Fig. 9-49 The completed porcelain fused to metal crown is placed over an Endo-Post dowel-core in a badly broken down lateral incisor.

References

1. Bergman, M., Holmlund, L. and Wictorin, L.: Noble metal alloy wires in cast posts. Mechanical properties and microstructure. *Odont Revy,* 25:273–287, 1974.

2. Charlton, G.: A prefabricated post and core for porcelain jacket crowns. *Brit Dent J,* 119:452–456, Nov. 1965.

3. Christy, J. M. and Pipko, D. J.: Fabrication of a dual-post veneer crown. *JADA,* 75:1419–1425, Dec. 1967.

4. Gerstein, H. and Burnell, S. C.: Prefabricated precision dowels. *JADA,* 69:787–791, Jun. 1964.

5. Harty, F. J.: A post crown technique using a nickel-cobalt chromium post. *Brit Dent J,* 132:394–399, May 1972.

6. Gruenwald, S.: The management of endodontically treated anterior teeth for jacket crowns. *Dent Dig,* 73:170–172, Apr. 1967.

7. Healey, H. J.: Coronal restoration of the pulpless tooth. *Dent Clin N Amer,* 1:885–896, Nov. 1957.

8. Sheets, C. E.: Dowel and core foundations. *J Prosthet Dent,* 23:58–65, Jan. 1970.

9. Mitchell, P. S. and Blass, M. S.: A technique for restoring the pulpless tooth. *J Ga Dent Assoc,* 46:14–17, Summer 1972.

10. Gerstein, H. and Evanson, L.: Precision posts or dowels. *Ill Dent J,* 32:70–73, Feb. 1963.

11. Yuodelis, R. and Morrison, K.: Full coverage restoration of pulpless anterior and bicuspid teeth. *J Canad Dent Assoc,* 32:516–521, Sept. 1966.

Chapter 10

Prefabricated Dowel/Composite Resin Core

Perhaps the simplest and most efficient method for the fabrication of a dowel core restoration is the composite resin core in combination with a prefabricated stainless steel dowel. The entire procedure, from completion of the endodontic obturation through the finished crown preparation, can be accomplished in a single appointment.[1–4]

This system can be used successfully in a wide range of clinical situations. At one extreme, this type of dowel has been shown to significantly strengthen teeth with no coronal destruction other than the endodontic access preparation.[5] At the other end of the spectrum, the prefabricated dowel/composite resin core can be used to restore both anterior and posterior teeth that have little or no intact coronal tooth structure.

Composite resin is easily and quickly placed as a core material, and it has the added advantage of being completely polymerized within minutes, allowing work on the core preparation to progress immediately. Preparations on amalgam cores, on the other hand, often must be delayed until a subsequent appointment. In addition, the resin requires less bulk of core material, making it the material of choice for anterior teeth where there is often minimal space around the dowel.

The prefabricated dowel/composite resin core is adequate for the restoration of single anterior teeth. However, most anterior bridge abutments should have cast dowel-cores.[5] Many molars requiring crowns can also be restored with this system. Two or three dowels can usually be placed for resistance to obliquely directed forces, and there is typically room for a generous bulk of core material. On molars with excessive destruction of coronal tooth structure or with very deep finish lines, amalgam may be the material of choice rather than composite resin. The decision to use an amalgam core requires no change in the technique for placement of the prefabricated dowel. In complex situations where *all* of the coronal tooth structure is missing on a potential abutment tooth, the two-piece cast dowel-core is the preferred restoration.

The dowel portion of the dowel/composite resin core acts to resist any lateral forces placed on the crown.[6] Care is taken to extend the finish lines for the final restoration well below the composite core.[7-11] When this is done, the crown will grasp the tooth, creating a "ferrule effect" to resist any vertical forces.[6] Auxiliary pins should be used routinely to resist any rotational forces placed on the restoration. Studies have shown that the prefabricated dowel/composite resin core does not adequately resist torque without auxiliary pins.[12] In addition, there is some evidence that pins embedded in core material across a tooth may have a "buttressing effect" and resist splitting forces on the root.[13]

The prefabricated dowel/composite resin core can also be used to restore a previously crowned tooth that has been endodontically treated.[14, 15] The head of the dowel is trimmed to fit within the confines of the access preparation and the dowel is cemented. The space around the head is then restored with amalgam or composite. This might be the method of choice in teeth with severe undercuts in the canal that would make a cast dowel-inlay difficult to fabricate.

There are several prefabricated stainless steel dowels of both parallel-sided and tapered designs that are suitable for use with composite resin cores. The technique for all of these systems is virtually the same with only minor modifications in the method of canal instrumentation. They should all be used with auxiliary pins.

Variations on both the dowel and core aspects of this technique have been advocated. Composite resin cores have been used with a threaded dowel, the Kurer Crown Saver.[16] All composite dowel-cores with no metal dowel have been recommended,[11] and acrylic dowel-cores have been used in children's teeth.[17] Finally, the stainless steel dowel has been utilized with no core at all, employing a dowel-sleeve inside the crown to fit over the head of the dowel, which essentially serves as its own core.[18]

TABLE 10-1   **Comparison of Instrument Sizes**

Instrument	Diameter (mm.)									
	0.9	1.0	1.1	1.2	1.3	1.4	1.5	1.6	1.7	1.8
Peeso Reamer	2	–	3	–	4	–	5	–	6	–
Para-Post Drill	.036 in. Brown	.040 in. Yellow	–	.050 in. Red		–	.060 in. Black		.070 in. Green	

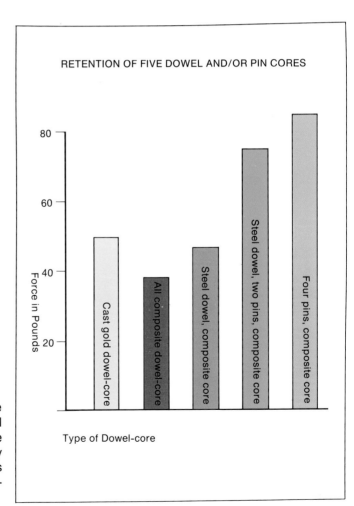

Fig. 10-1   The retention (tensile capacity) of the stainless steel dowel and composite resin core is superior to that exhibited by other types of dowel-cores tested. (Based on data by Newburg and Pameijer.[12])

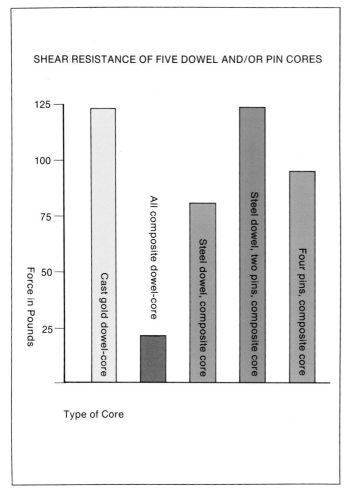

SHEAR RESISTANCE OF FIVE DOWEL AND/OR PIN CORES

125 —

100 —

75 —

50 —

25 —

Force in Pounds

Cast gold dowel-core

All composite dowel-core

Steel dowel, composite core

Steel dowel, two pins, composite core

Four pins, composite core

Type of Core

Fig. 10-2 Resistance to shear force shown by the stainless steel dowel and composite resin core is excellent. Special attention should be paid to the all composite resin dowel-core. Although it has moderate tensile strength, its resistance to shear force is quite poor. (Based on data by Newburg and Pameijer.[12])

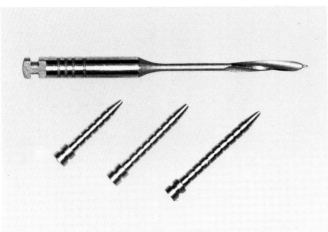

Fig. 10-3 The BCH system* is comprised of two or three lengths in each of five diameters, for a total of 14 sizes. They are meant to be used with Peeso reamers and they come in diameters of 0.8 mm., 1.0 mm., 1.2 mm., 1.4 mm., and 1.6 mm. The dowels are serrated and parallel-sided, with tapered tips and a round button on the occlusal end.

* BCH, Unitek Corp., Monrovia, CA.

Fig. 10-4 The C · I (Calibrated Instrument) Kit* utilizes three rotary instruments for the dowel preparation. The preparation is started with a bibevel twist drill, enlarged with a pointed reamer, and finished with a special tapered fissure bur. The corrugated stainless steel dowels have a taper of 2.6° and are available in two diameters: 1.0–1.4 mm. and 1.2–1.7 mm. The smaller number represents the diameter at the tip, while the larger number is the diameter 10 mm. from the tip. There is a separate set of instruments for each dowel size.

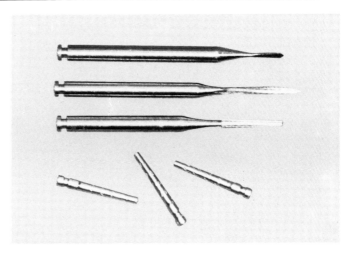

* C · I Kit, Parkell, Farmingdale, NY.

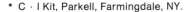

Fig. 10-5 Colorama* dowels were meant to be used for fabricating temporary crowns, but they can be used with auxiliary pins and composite resin cores. The tips display an average taper of 6.2°, while the bodies of the smooth dowels are parallel-sided. The canal is enlarged with a color-coded combination tapered/parallel reamer of matching size. The size ranges (tip diameter and diameter 10 mm. from the tip) are 0.8–1.3 mm., 0.9–1.4 mm., 1.0–1.6 mm., 1.0–1.8 mm., and 1.1–2.0 mm.

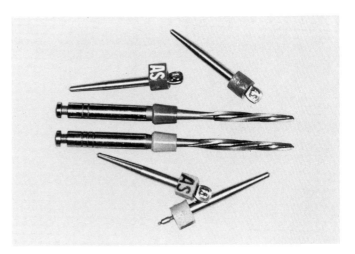

* Colorama, J. Aderer Inc. (Metaux Precieux), Long Island City, NY.

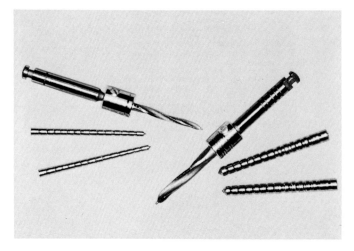

Fig. 10-6 Ellman NuBond Fast Posts* are serrated stainless steel dowels with a 1.6° taper. The canal is prepared with tapered reamers of matching sizes. There are six sizes: 0.9–1.2 mm., 1.1–1.4 mm., 1.3–1.6 mm., 1.5–1.8 mm., 1.7–2.1 mm., and 1.9–2.3 mm.

* NuBond Fast Post, Ellman Dent Mfg. Co., Hewlett, NY.

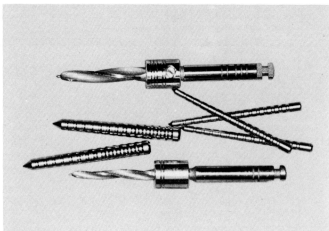

Fig. 10-7 The P-D Crown Post* is also a stainless steel serrated dowel. It has a 1.6° taper and comes in six sizes: 0.9–1.3 mm., 1.1–1.5 mm., 1.3–1.7 mm., 1.5–1.9 mm., 1.7–2.1 mm., and 1.9–2.3 mm. The dowel preparation is accomplished with tapered engine reamers.

* P-D Crown Post, Union Broach Corp., Long Island City, NY.

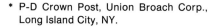

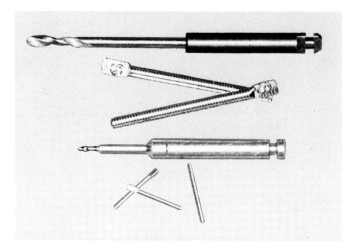

Fig. 10-8 The Para-Post* is a serrated, parallel-sided, stainless steel dowel which is used with a large color-coded twist drill of matching size. The dowels are available in five diameters: 0.9 mm., 1.0 mm., 1.25 mm., 1.50 mm., and 1.75 mm. Auxiliary pin holes for Minim pins are placed in the root face with a 0.5 mm. Kodex drill. Para-Post is also available in a tapered-end parallel-sided dowel.

* Para-Post, Whaledent International, New York, NY.

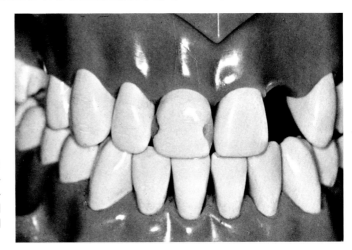

Fig. 10-9 The typical indication for a prefabricated dowel/composite resin core is an endodontically treated maxillary central incisor with large existing mesial and distal restorations.

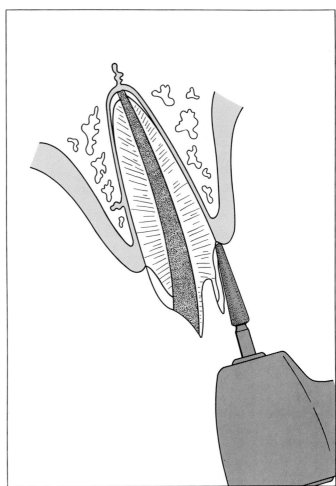

Fig. 10-10 The coronal preparation for a prefabricated dowel/composite resin core is accomplished in much the same way as it is for a custom cast dowel-core.

233

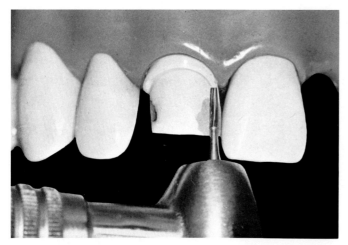

Fig. 10-11   The incisal and axial surfaces are reduced as they would be for a typical preparation for an anterior porcelain fused to metal crown. A facial shoulder 1.25 mm. wide is established, but it is not necessarily carried into the sulcus at this time.

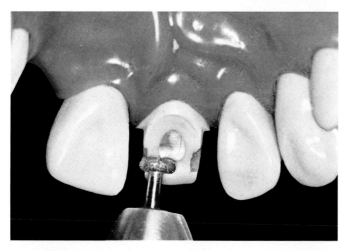

Fig. 10-12   The lingual reduction is accomplished with a wheel diamond. An effort should be made to gain adequate reduction and still maintain a vertical lingual wall on the preparation.

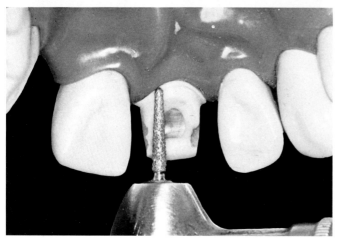

Fig. 10-13   The lingual finish line is prepared with a round-end tapered diamond. If the lingual wall is too short, a shoulder is carried around the lingual to establish adequate length. Up to this point, all existing restorations and cements have been ignored, and the preparation is more or less ideal.

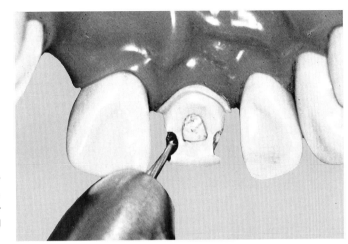

Fig. 10-14 All existing restorations and caries are removed. Any questionable or stained dentin should be excavated, leaving only sound tooth structure.

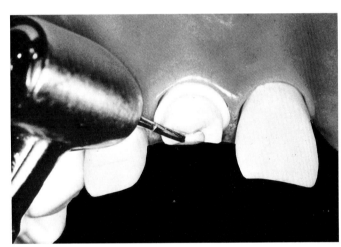

Fig. 10-15 Any unsupported or undercut areas are now eliminated. No effort should be made to save thin or questionable dentinal walls. At least two flat areas with adequate bulk of tooth structure should be prepared to accommodate pins.

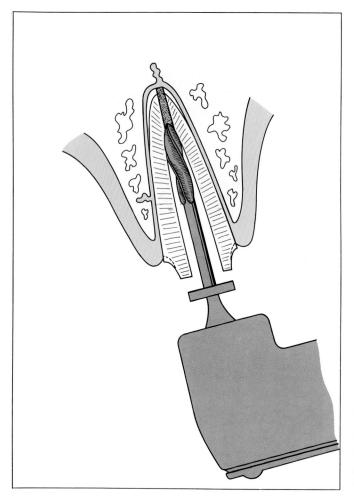

Fig. 10-16 At this point, the preparation of the canal space is initiated. Some of the gutta percha in the coronal portion of the canal can be removed with a hot instrument. The length is established with a Peeso reamer or a Gates Glidden drill.

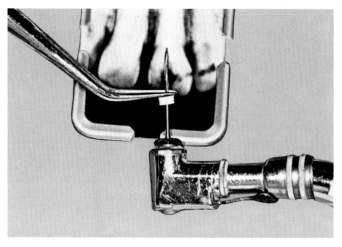

Fig. 10-17 The length of the dowel space is measured. Every effort is made to prepare the canal space to a length equal to or greater than that of the final crown. The space should be as long as possible without encroaching on the 4.0 mm. apical seal.

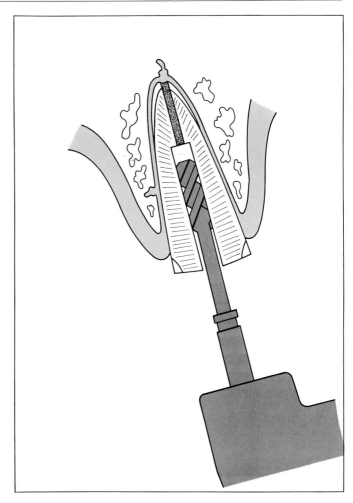

Fig. 10-18 The shaping of the canal is now accomplished with the Para-Post drill.

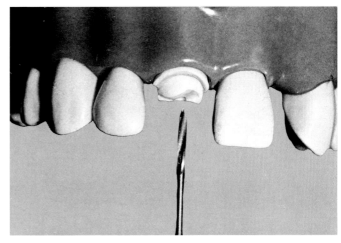

Fig. 10-19 The dowel space preparation can be started with either a Peeso reamer or a Para-Post twist drill whose diameter is smaller than that of the final dowel size (see Table 10-1). Continue to increase the diameter of the reamers until the desired size is reached.

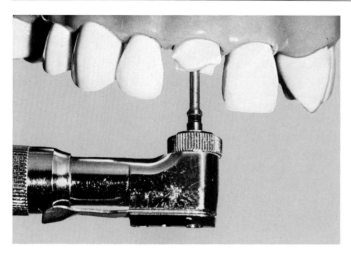

Fig. 10-20 The drill which will produce the final diameter should be used to prepare the entire length of the canal. A minimum number of insertions should be made with the drill, since many retentive failures of prefabricated dowels are caused by overinstrumentation of the canal.

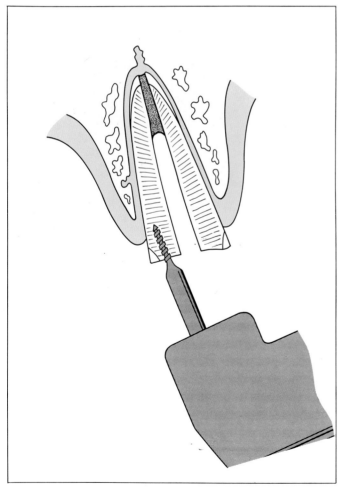

Fig. 10-21 Pin holes are drilled around the canal space so that auxiliary pins can be placed.

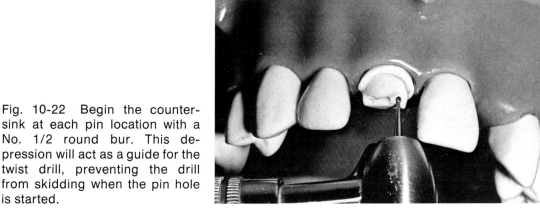

Fig. 10-22 Begin the countersink at each pin location with a No. 1/2 round bur. This depression will act as a guide for the twist drill, preventing the drill from skidding when the pin hole is started.

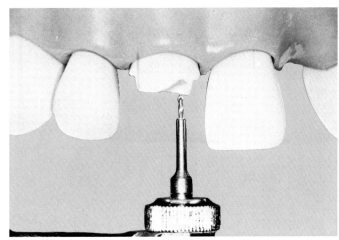

Fig. 10-23 The pin holes are drilled to a depth of 2 mm. with a self-limiting 0.5 mm. twist drill. It is not necessary for these pin holes to parallel the canal.

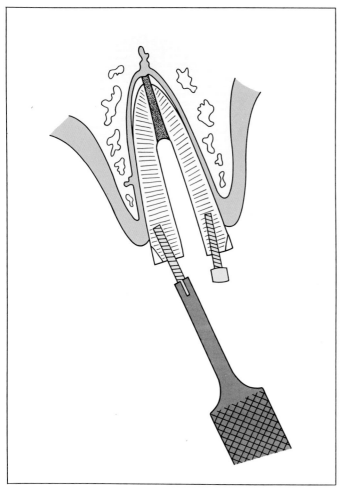

Fig. 10-24 The pins can now be placed. In this example, self-threading pins were used. Cemented pins are preferred by some authors because self-threading pins do produce stress, and they can cause dentinal crazing. For this reason, there is some opposition to their use in endodontically treated teeth.[19] If there is adequate bulk of tooth structure, and if the tooth has been nonvital for only a short period of time so that resilience is not impaired, small threaded pins should not represent too great a hazard.

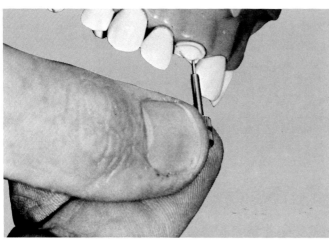

Fig. 10-25 A hand wrench is used in an easily accessible area. When the pins are threaded into place, stop as soon as any resistance is encountered to prevent dentinal fracture. "Back off" slightly to reduce stress, but not enough to produce a loose fit. The pins are shortened, if needed, to insure that they will be within the confines of the completed preparation and that they will not interfere with placement of the dowel. At least 2.0 mm. of pin should be left exposed.

Fig. 10-26 The stainless steel dowel is now tried into the prepared space. Any reduction in length should be accomplished from the apical end, as the dowel head can provide added retention to the core material. The dowel should have a snug fit in the canal. If it does not, the canal has been overinstrumented.

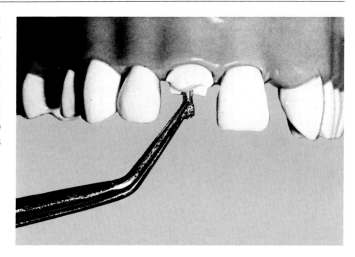

Fig. 10-27 A thin mix of cement is made. Although zinc phosphate is used here, no difference in retentive ability has been found among zinc phosphate, polycarboxylate, and glass ionomer cements.[20, 21]

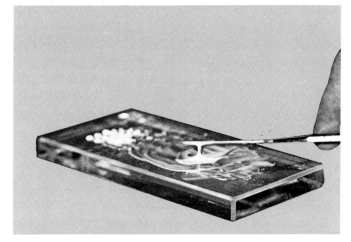

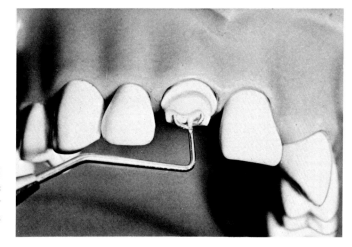

Fig. 10-28 Cement is placed into the canal. An endodontic plugger, periodontal probe, or Lentulo spiral can be used for this purpose.

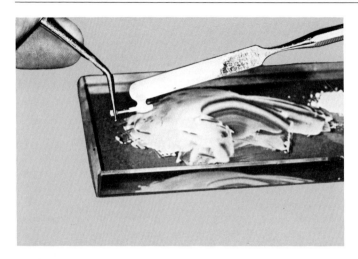

Fig. 10-29   A generous layer of cement is placed on the dowel. The Para-post dowel has a cement vent down its entire length, so preparation of this feature is not necessary.

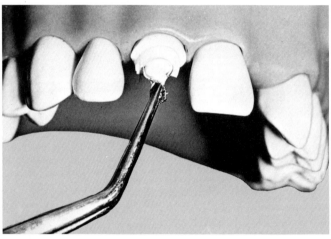

Fig. 10-30   The dowel is slowly pushed to the end of the canal space, allowing time for excess cement to escape. Hold the dowel in place with finger pressure until the initial cement set occurs.

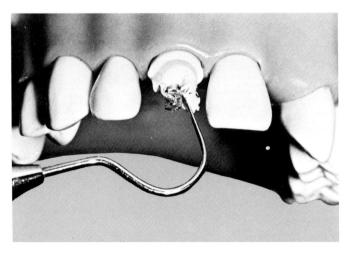

Fig. 10-31   After the cement has achieved its initial set, excess is removed from around the pins and the coronal portion of the dowel.

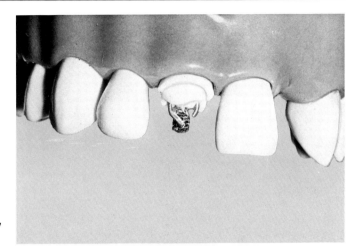

Fig. 10-32 The tooth is now ready for core fabrication.

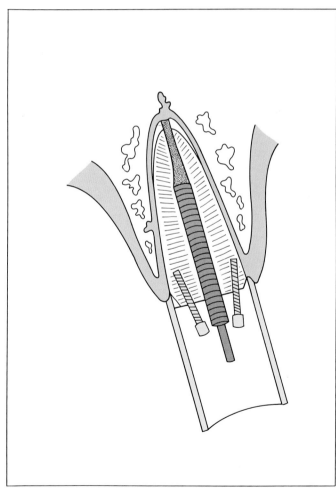

Fig. 10-33 A matrix band or crown form is placed around the tooth to permit the placement of composite resin.

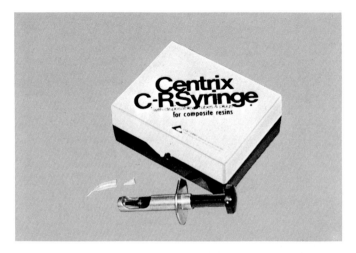

Fig. 10-34 The Centrix syringe* is effective in placing resin around the pins and dowel and eliminates the possibility of voids in the core.

* Centrix C-R Syringe, Centrix Inc., Stratford, CT.

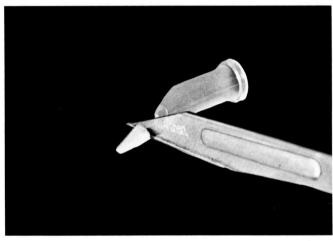

Fig. 10-35 The syringe tip has a restricted end with a small lumen designed for injecting resin into small Class III cavity preparations. For placing a core, it is necessary to remove a large segment of the plastic tip with a sharp knife. This produces a wider aperture to accommodate the bulk of resin necessary to make the typical core.

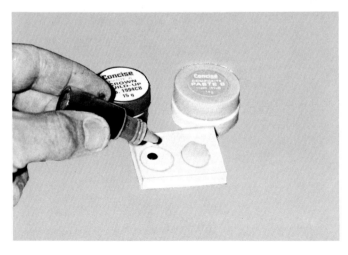

Fig. 10-36 The composite material should contrast in color with the tooth.[8, 9] A small drop of green food coloring is added to the resin to achieve a marked contrast.

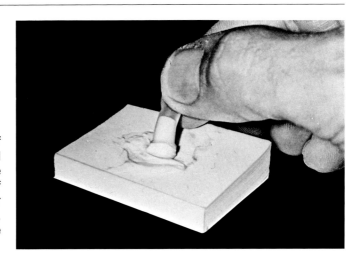

Fig. 10-37 A sizable bulk of composite resin is mixed and loaded into the syringe tip. A core requires a much larger mix of resin than is normally used for Class III restorations. In addition, not all of the material can be expressed from the syringe.

Fig. 10-38 The conical rubber plunger is placed in the syringe tip behind the composite resin, and the tip is inserted through the hole in the end of the syringe. Push the plunger until some material is extruded to confirm a free flow of resin.

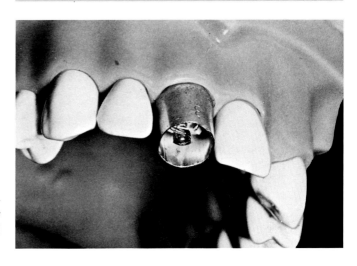

Fig. 10-39 A copper band matrix which has been previously trimmed and fitted is placed around the tooth.

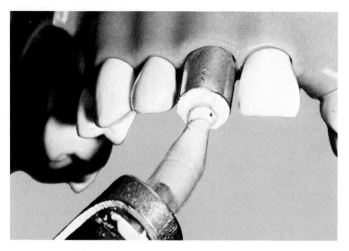

Fig. 10-40 The composite resin is injected carefully, but quickly, around the dowel head and the pins. The matrix is then filled to overflowing, avoiding air entrapment within the core.

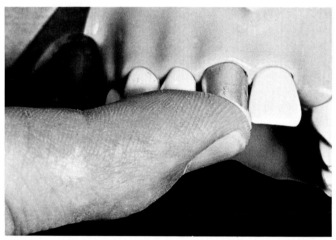

Fig. 10-41 Firmly place a fingertip over the open end of the copper band to compress the composite resin and keep the matrix stable as the material polymerizes.

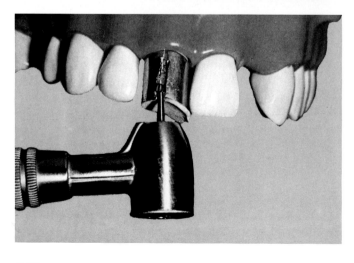

Fig. 10-42 When the resin has cured completely, the matrix is split with a high speed round bur and removed.

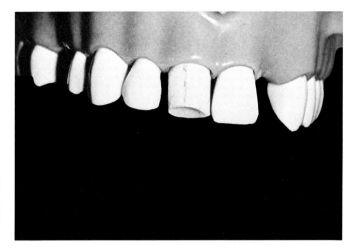

Fig. 10-43 The resulting composite resin build-up is a very dense, cylindrical blank from which a crown preparation can be shaped.

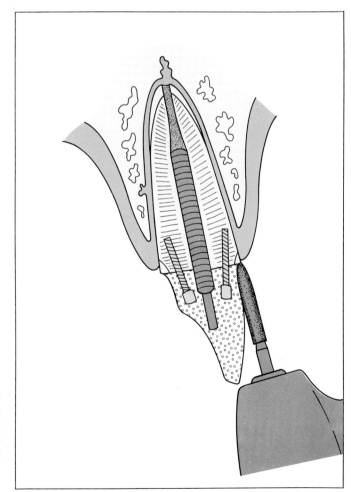

Fig. 10-44 A preparation for a porcelain fused to metal crown is accomplished with diamond stones in a high speed handpiece, treating the composite resin as though it were tooth structure.

247

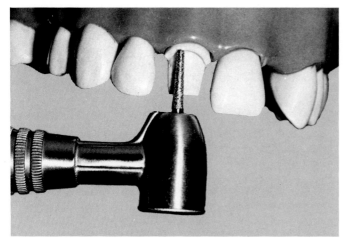

Fig. 10-45 Special attention is paid to placing all the crown preparation finish lines well below the margin of the core. Axial reduction for construction of the porcelain fused to metal crown should be generous, since there is no reason to be overly conservative.

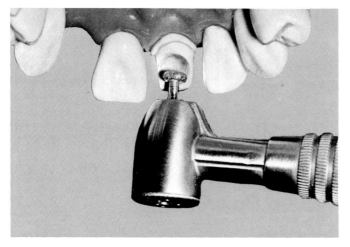

Fig. 10-46 Lingual reduction consists of a concave cingulum and a short vertical lingual wall.

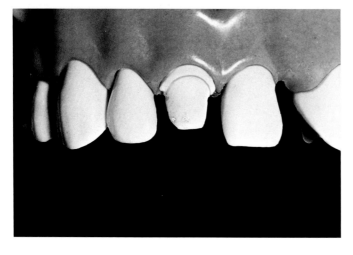

Fig. 10-47 The completed preparation in the composite resin core as viewed from the facial.

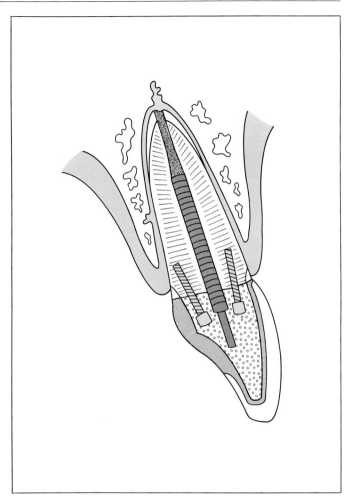

Fig. 10-48 The porcelain fused to metal crown can now be fabricated over the composite resin core, which is retained and bolstered by a stainless steel dowel.

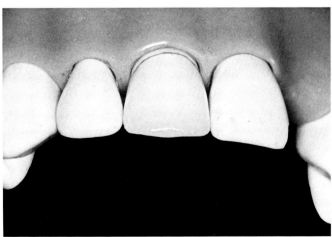

Fig. 10-49 The completed porcelain fused to metal restoration.

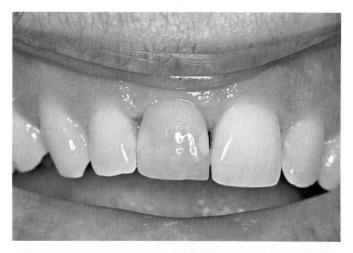

Fig. 10-50 This patient presented with a discolored endodontically treated maxillary incisor
with large mesial and distal resin
restorations.

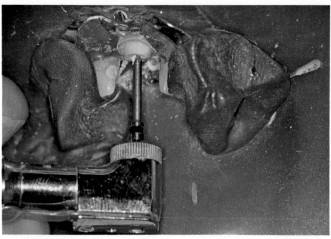

Fig. 10-51 After the coronal
preparation had been accomplished, the dowel space was
completed with a twist drill.

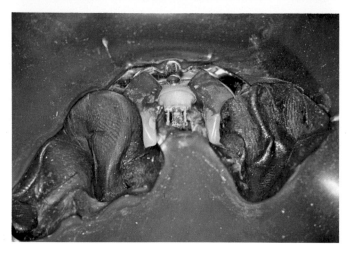

Fig. 10-52 The prefabricated
stainless steel Para-Post and two
pins have been placed.

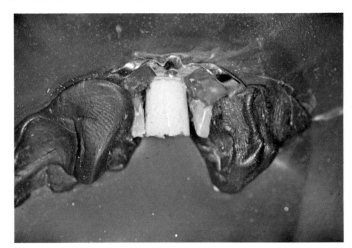

Fig. 10-53 The composite resin core is seen after the copper band had been removed.

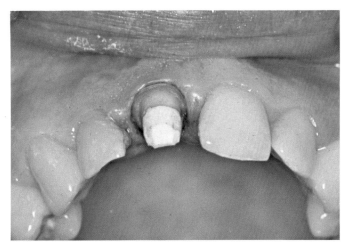

Fig. 10-54 The extensions of the opaque white composite core are easily seen in the completed preparation. Tissue had been retracted for the impression.

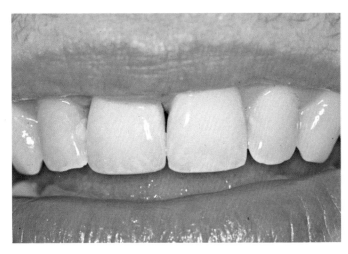

Fig. 10-55 The finished porcelain fused to metal crown.

References

1. Baum, L.: Dowel placement in the endodontically treated tooth. *J Conn St Dent Assoc,* 53:116–117, Summer 1979.

2. Ram, Z.: T-pins in a direct pattern technique for posts and cores. *J Prosthet Dent,* 40:103–106, Jul. 1978.

3. Sherman, J. A.: One visit post and core technique. *Dent Surv,* 52:40–41, May 1976.

4. Spalten, R. G.: Composite resins to restore mutilated teeth. *J Prosthet Dent,* 25:323–326, Mar. 1971.

5. Kantor, M. E. and Pines, M. S.: A comparative study of restorative techniques for pulpless teeth. *J Prosthet Dent,* 38:405–412, Oct. 1977.

6. Steele, G. D.: Reinforced composite resin foundations. *J Prosthet Dent,* 30:816–819, Nov. 1973.

7. Baraban, D. J.: Immediate restoration of pulpless teeth. *J Prosthet Dent,* 28:607–612, Dec. 1972.

8. Federick, D. R.: A one-appointment dowel and core technic. *Dent Surv,* 52:50–51, Dec. 1976.

9. Schmidt, J. R., Ehrenkranz, H., Mohamed, S. E. and Franklin, M. E.: A single visit post and core procedure. *NY St Dent J,* 39:604–610, Dec. 1973.

10. Spanauf, A. J.: Dowel and core foundations using the composite Adaptic. *Quint Int,* 3:45–47, Sept. 1972.

11. Stahl, G. J. and O'Neal, R. B.: The composite resin dowel and core. *J Prosthet Dent,* 33:642–648, Jun. 1975.

12. Newburg, R. E. and Pameijer, C. H.: Retentive properties of post and core systems. *J Prosthet Dent,* 36:636–643, Dec. 1976.

13. Watson, R. J.: Amalgam foundations for anterior teeth. *Dent Dig,* 73:206–207, May 1967.

14. Federick, D. R.: An application of the dowel and composite resin core technique. *J Prosthet Dent,* 32:420–423, Oct. 1974.

15. Federick, D. R.: Secondary intention dowel and core. *J Prosthet Dent,* 34:41–47, Jul. 1975.

16. Kurer, P. F. and Kurer, H. G.: The Kurer crown saver. A method of restoration of multi-rooted endodontically treated teeth. *Quint Int,* 8:29–33, Feb. 1977.

17. Harris, W. E.: A method of non-metal post/core retention for crowns. *J Ga Dent Assoc,* 50:19–21, Feb. 1977.

18. Whiteside, W. D.: A simplified dowel crown technique. *J Prosthet Dent,* 23:554–559, May 1970.

19. Caputo, A. A. and Standlee, J. P.: Pins and posts–why, when and how. *Dent Clin N Amer,* 20:299–311, Apr. 1976.

20. Hanson, E. C. and Caputo, A. A.: Cementing mediums and retentive characteristics. *J Prosthet Dent,* 32:551–557, Nov. 1974.

21. Krupp, J. D., Caputo, A. A., Trabert, K. C. and Standlee, J. P.: Dowel retention with glass ionomer cement. *J Prosthet Dent,* 41:163–166, Feb. 1979.

Chapter 11

Parallel Threaded Dowel (Pretapped)

There is another type of dowel which permits the completion of the tooth build-up in a single appointment. It employs threads on its parallel sides for retention, and it is inserted into a canal whose walls are prethreaded with a special tap.* It differs from other types of dowels because it is not passively inserted into the canal and held in place entirely by the cement. Whether this threaded dowel is retained by mechanical interaction, or simply by increasing the surface area two or threefold,[1] it demonstrates superior retention to other types of dowels. It was found to be 2.0 to 3.4 times as retentive as parallel serrated dowels in one study,[2] and 5.0 times as retentive in another.[3]

Threaded dowels are not without controversy, however. Concern has been expressed over increasing the potential of root fracture by threading dowels into the canal.[4-7] The stresses generated by threaded dowels certainly are greater than those generated by dowels retained by cement alone.[8, 9] However, mechanical testing has shown that when the tap is used properly, fracture cannot be induced.[10] Frequent cleaning of the tap is essential to reduce stress and prevent resultant root fracture.[9-11]

As with any threaded retention device, there is some hazard for the tooth. The risk is minimal if the tooth in which it is to be placed is properly selected and if the dowel is used correctly. The Kurer Anchor should not be used on teeth with thin, fragile walls, nor should it be used by the heavy-handed operator (a condition least likely to be recognized by the one who most needs to know, unfortunately).

* Kurer Crown Anchor, Teledyne Getz, Elk Grove Village, IL.

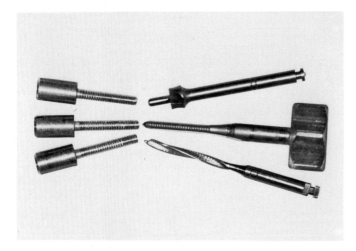

Fig. 11-1 The original crown anchor consists of a stainless steel threaded shank (dowel) with a slotted machine brass head (core).[12] The canal is enlarged with an elongated engine reamer, and its orifice is countersunk with a root facer. A tap is then used to thread the canal for insertion of the anchor.

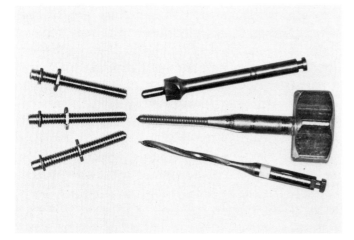

Fig. 11-2 The Kurer Fin-lock utilizes a threaded "root face fin" or lock nut to snug against the countersunk root face.[13] A narrow collar near the slotted end serves as additional retention for the composite resin core which will be added after cementation of the anchor. All other instruments used are the same as those used for the crown anchor.

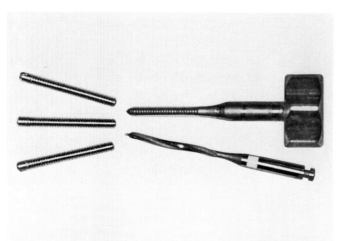

Fig. 11-3 The Kurer Crown Saver is a simple threaded dowel that has neither a head nor a lock nut and, therefore, does not require the use of a root facing instrument. It consists of a parallel threaded dowel which is cemented in the canal and serves as the retention for a composite resin build-up.[14, 15] This technique is very similar to that of the serrated steel dowels used with composite cores (see Chapter 10).

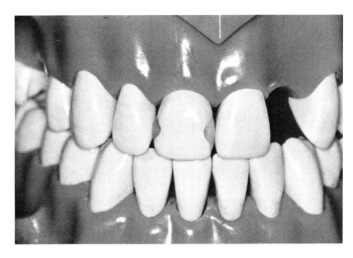

Fig. 11-4 The parallel threaded anchor can be used in the restoration of any tooth with sufficient bulk of root structure to support it. However, because it does require removal of nearly all coronal tooth structure, its use should ideally be reserved for those teeth with extensive destruction of coronal tooth structure.

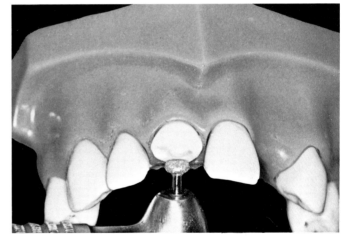

Fig. 11-5 Preparation of the tooth for this type of anchor is started by removal of all tooth structure to within 0.5 mm. of the gingiva.[16] This is most easily accomplished through the use of a small wheel diamond.

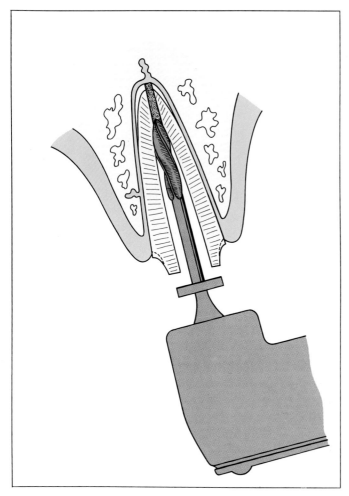

Fig. 11-6 Preparation of the dowel space will be accomplished with an engine reamer which resembles the Peeso reamer, except for the greater length of the cutting flutes (15 mm., compared with 8.0 mm. for a No. 6 Peeso reamer).

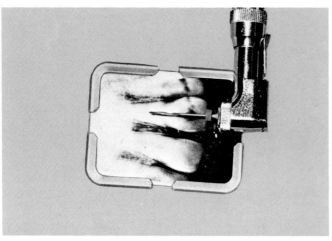

Fig. 11-7 Compare the reamer with a radiograph of the tooth being restored. Place a rubber stop on the reamer to provide a reference mark for depth of penetration.

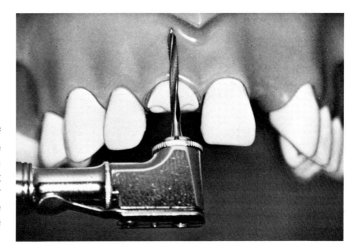

Fig. 11-8 Use Peeso reamers of increasing diameter to provide the initial enlargement and length of the dowel preparation. Do not use a Peeso reamer that is larger than the Kurer reamer for the corresponding anchor (see Table 11-1).

TABLE 11-1 **Comparison of Reamer Sizes**

	Diameter (mm.)						
Reamer	1.1	1.3	1.4	1.5	1.6	1.7	1.8
Peeso	No. 3	No. 4	–	No. 5	–	No. 6	–
Kurer	–	No. 0	No. 1	–	No. 2	–	No. 3

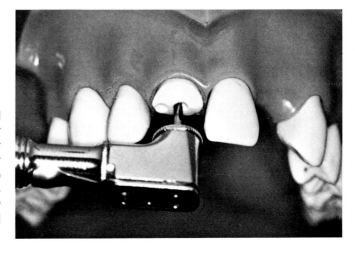

Fig. 11-9 Complete the dowel preparation with the reamer which matches the size of anchor selected. Too small a reamer could lead to tooth fracture. Too large a reamer or overinstrumentation with the correct size reamer produces an oversized canal with poor retention.[11]

257

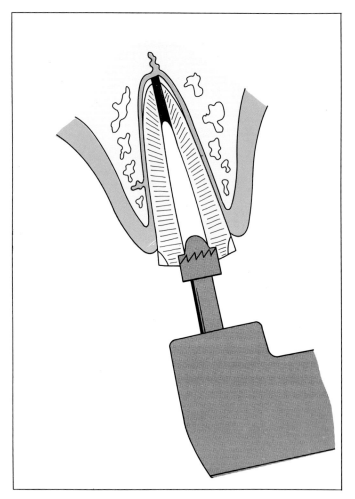

Fig. 11-10   A root facer is used to provide a flat countersink on the root surface around the mouth of the canal. The countersink allows the head, or core, of the anchor to be set completely within tooth structure, providing resistance to obliquely directed forces.[17] It provides protection to the head and makes it less susceptible to fracture.[18]

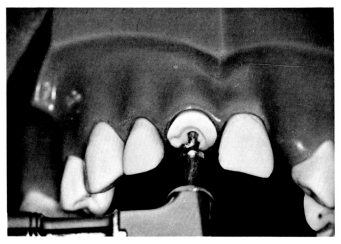

Fig. 11-11   Insert the noncutting spigot of the root facer into the orifice of the canal. Be sure that the axis of the countersink and, therefore, the shaft of the root facer are coincident with the axis of the dowel preparation. Failure to observe this simple precaution could result in extremely high stress concentrations.[9]

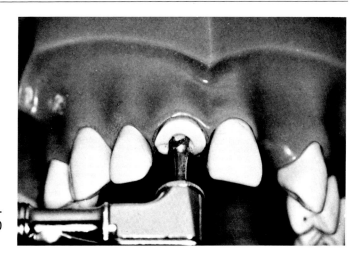

Fig. 11-12 Prepare the counter-sink to a minimum depth of 1.0 mm.

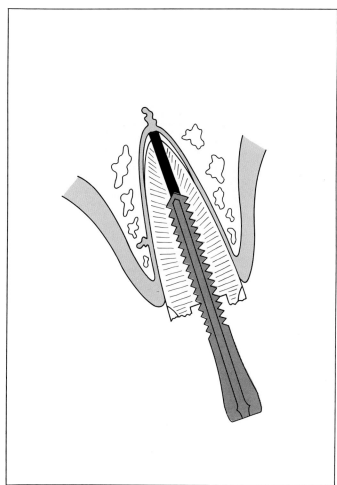

Fig. 11-13 Use the tap to thread the canals. Because this is the time of greatest stress build-up, it must be done carefully. Use only new, sharp taps. A tap should be discarded when the anchors in its kit have been used up.

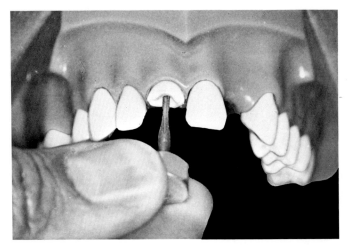

Fig. 11-14 Use gentle finger pressure when rotating the tap. Stop when *any* resistance is encountered. Keep the canal moist to lubricate the tap. Make no more than two revolutions of the tap in a clockwise direction, and then remove the tap.[9]

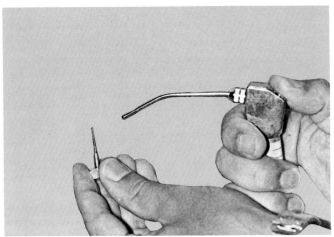

Fig. 11-15 Every time the tap is removed from the canal, clean it off with spray from the water-air syringe. Removing debris from the threads of the tap is extremely important in the prevention of damaging stresses while the canal is being threaded. When the threading is completed, irrigate the canal thoroughly to remove as much debris as possible.

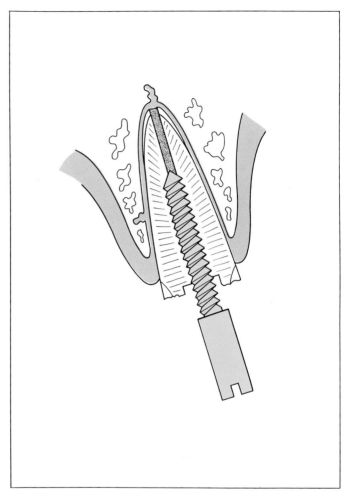

Fig. 11-16 The anchor is tried in to establish its length and determine the adjustment necessary in the length of the dowel.

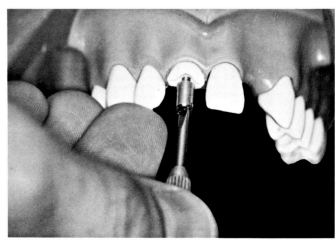

Fig. 11-17 The anchor driver, a small screwdriver, is placed in the short head to thread the anchor into the canal. Stop as soon as resistance is encountered, because stress is developed when the dowel "bottoms out."

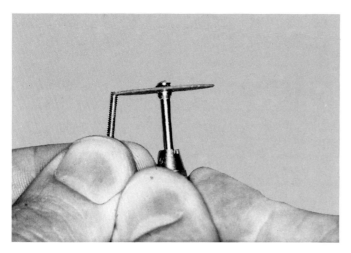

Fig. 11-18 Measure the length of threaded dowel between the base of the core and the countersunk root face, or count the rows of threads which are showing in the same area. Use a 7/8 inch Carborundum disc to cut off a corresponding length at the end of the dowel. Thread the dowel back into the canal to verify that sufficient length has been removed. Again, do not overtorque the anchor when it reaches the apical end of the dowel preparation.

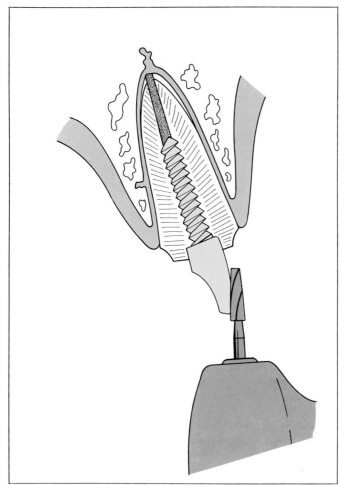

Fig. 11-19 The head, or core, of the anchor must be shaped to resemble the contours of a crown preparation for the final restoration. Four adjustments are usually required: (1) The incisal edge will probably need to be shortened; (2) the incisal portion of the facial surface must be reduced to move the inciso-facial line angle to the lingual; (3) a concave area in the incisal 2/3 of the lingual surface must be created; and (4) the axial walls should be slightly tapered. While this can be accomplished on the tooth after the anchor has been cemented, it is uncomfortable for the patient and time-consuming as well. In addition, wear and tear on cutting instruments can be considerable.

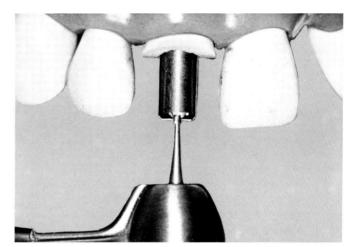

Fig. 11-20 Thread the anchor into the tooth until it is firmly seated. With a small round bur or a No. 34 inverted cone, mark the desired length of the incisal edge on the facial surface of the head.

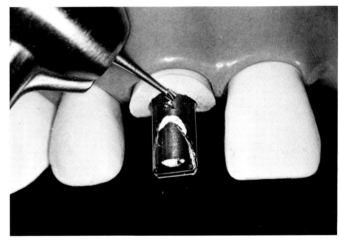

Fig. 11-21 Trace the proximal and incisal extensions of the in-ciso-facial plane which are needed to move the incisal portion of the facial surface back into harmony with the facial surfaces of the adjacent teeth. Imprint the midpoint of the surface with a distinctive mark which will be easily identifiable after the anchor is removed from the tooth.

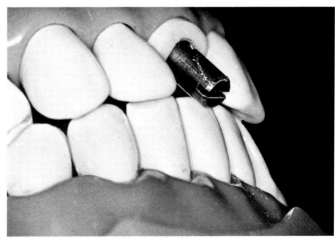

Fig. 11-22 Examine the lingual and incisal areas of the tooth when the patient's teeth are in occlusion in order to estimate the extensions and depth of the lingual concavity.

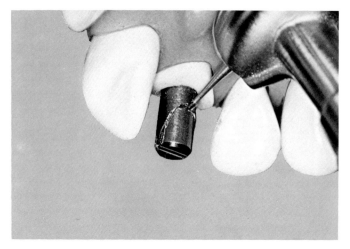

Fig. 11-23 Use the same bur to mark the proximal and gingival extensions of the lingual concavity. Place another distinctive mark in the middle of the lingual surface, apical to the concavity, to assist in orienting the core once it has been removed from the mouth.

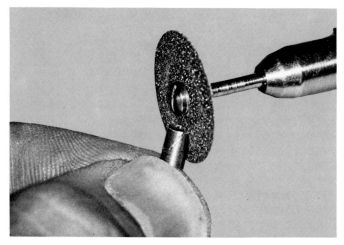

Fig. 11-24 Cut off the excess incisal length and flatten the incisofacial plane with a Carborundum separating disc. Extend the plane to the outline cut on the core when it was on the tooth. Because of the heat generated by the grinding, it will probably be necessary to hold the dowel with a wet towel, or to dip the core in water frequently.

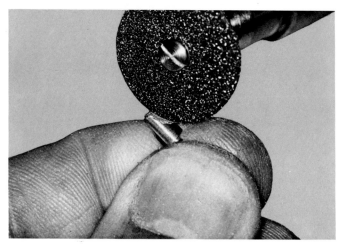

Fig. 11-25 Use the disc to hollow grind the large concavity in the incisal 2/3 of the lingual surface. The brass head should now be assuming the configuration of a crown preparation.

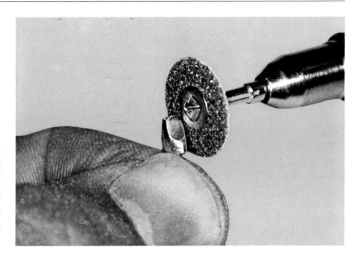

Fig. 11-26 Since the parallel sides of the core will present problems in the fabrication and seating of the porcelain fused to metal crown, a slight taper is added to the axial wall with a coarse garnet disc.

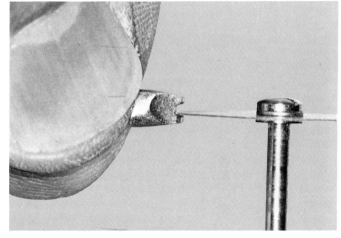

Fig. 11-27 In all likelihood, the previous steps will have eliminated much or all of the slot in the brass head. It must be restored in order to screw the anchor into the tooth during cementation. The Carborundum disc is used to cut a slot at right angles to the incisal edge.

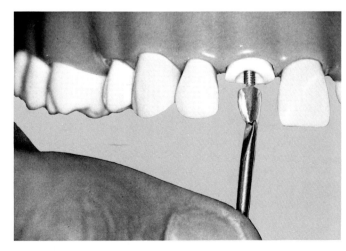

Fig. 11-28 Thread the anchor back into the tooth to verify that there is enough reduction in the inciso-facial area to allow the fabrication of an esthetic restoration. Check for adequate clearance with the opposing teeth. Make any required adjustments and proceed with cementation.

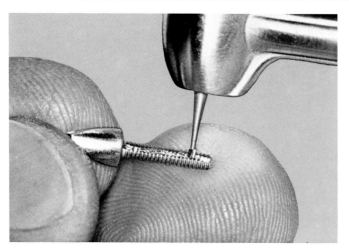

Fig. 11-29 A cement escape vent is extremely important in the seating of a threaded dowel. Cut a large v-shaped groove from the apical end of the dowel to the base of the core.

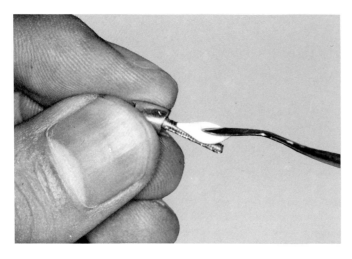

Fig. 11-30 Prepare a thin mix of zinc phosphate cement on a glass slab and apply a thin, uniform coat over the dowel. Do not place any cement into the canal. Cement does not play a significant role in the retention of the threaded dowel, but it is important as a sealer. Because of the extremely close fit of the dowel in the threaded canal, it is difficult to express the excess cement without producing a strong hydraulic effect. Large quantities of cement would make it impossible to seat the dowel completely.

Fig. 11-31 Insert the dowel in the canal and thread it to position with the screwdriver. Stop from time to time to allow excess cement to escape from the vent. If the dowel tends to overseat (i.e., turn past the position at which the facial and lingual features are in proper alignment) do not hesitate to reverse the anchor 1/8 or 1/4 turn to produce correct alignment. Stress generation is probably less severe when the countersink is not fully engaged anyway.[9]

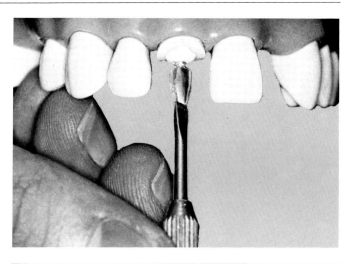

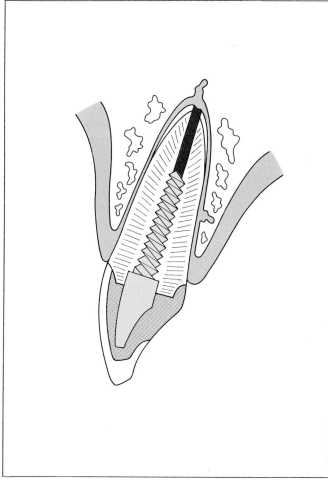

Fig. 11-32 When the cement has set, the tooth which has been built up with the Kurer crown anchor is ready for fabrication of the final restoration.

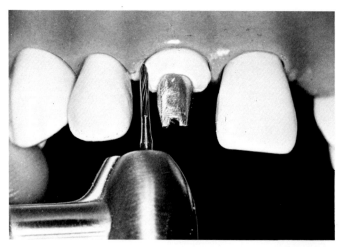

Fig. 11-33 The nature of the initial tooth preparation leaves a wide shoulder completely surrounding the core. If a porcelain jacket crown is to be employed, it is necessary only to smooth the shoulder and make sure that it is far enough subgingival to hide the margin. If a porcelain fused to metal crown is to be employed, it will be necessary to place a narrow bevel around the preparation, using a chamfer bur.*

* No. 282 010, Brasseler USA, Inc., Savannah, GA.

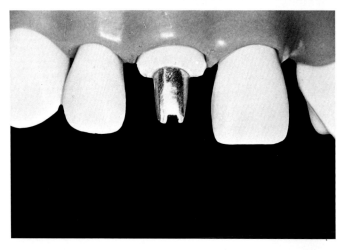

Fig. 11-34 The completed preparation is ready for an impression. Although the shoulder is a little wider than usual, the core resembles a crown preparation in other respects. The incisal slot could present a problem during the making of the impression or the fabrication of the coping. The small projection on each side would form acute internal angles in the coping wax pattern which could trap bubbles during investing. The resulting nodules in the casting would prevent complete seating.

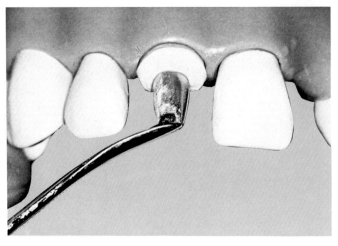

Fig. 11-35 Therefore, the slot is filled in with soft wax or cement for the impression.

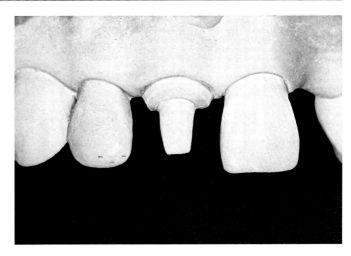

Fig. 11-36 The cast made from the impression portrays an ideal preparation with an intact incisal edge. Although the slot could be blocked out on the cast, it could be a problem if a separate working cast and master die are used. When it is blocked out on the core in the mouth, these problems are eliminated.

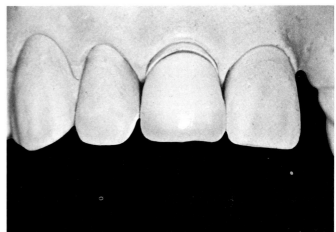

Fig. 11-37 Fabrication of the restoration on the working cast is carried out in the usual manner.

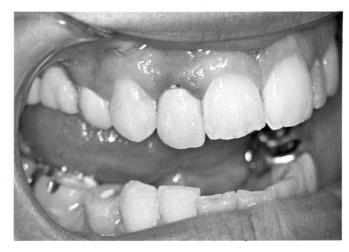

Fig. 11-38 This maxillary lateral incisor had been restored with a crown which relied on four pins, each approximately 2 mm. in length, as its sole means of retention. The crown had failed.

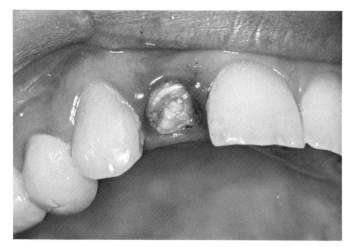

Fig. 11-39 Examination of the root stump revealed a tooth with no coronal tooth structure. However, there was good bulk of tooth structure around the root canal. This was an ideal indication for the use of a Kurer Crown Anchor.

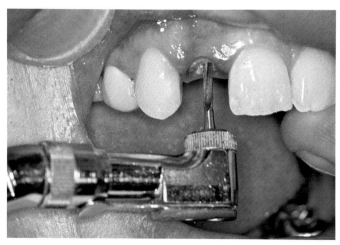

Fig. 11-40 A dowel preparation had been done at the time of the endodontic treatment. It was merely enlarged at this time with the appropriate reamer for the Kurer Anchor.

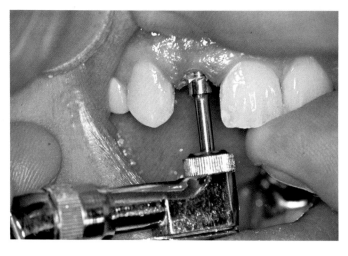

Fig. 11-41 The root face surrounding the orifice of the root canal was countersunk with the root facer.

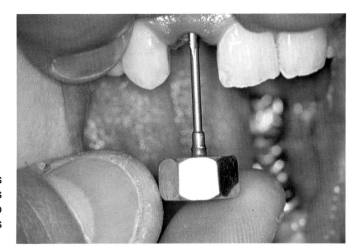

Fig. 11-42 The canal was threaded with a tap, which was removed after every two turns to clean the tooth debris from its threads.

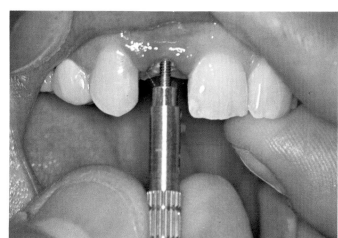

Fig. 11-43 The anchor was inserted with the screwdriver provided with the kit.

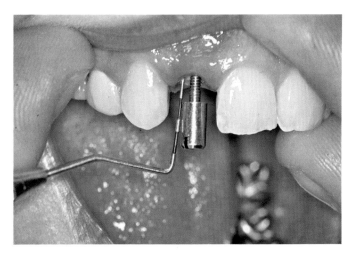

Fig. 11-44 The length of dowel by which the head of the anchor was lifted from the root face was determined by use of a periodontal probe.

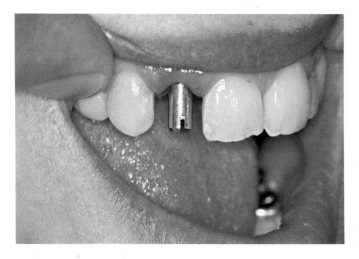

Fig. 11-45 After the excess length had been removed, the anchor was tried in again. It was now marked for modification.

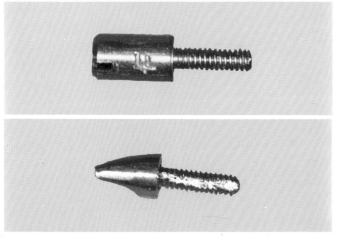

Fig. 11-46 The anchor with intact brass core (head) is shown above. In the lower view, the modifications of the core have been completed and it is ready for cementation.

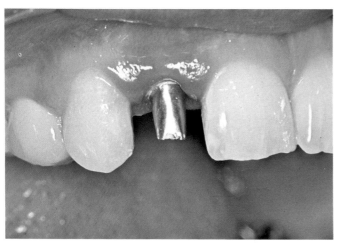

Fig. 11-47 The completed anchor is seen after cementation. The incisal slot has been filled in to facilitate the fabrication of the final crown.

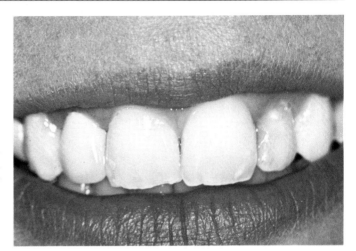

Fig. 11-48 The completed porcelain fused to metal crown has been cemented over the Kurer Anchor to complete the restoration of a tooth which was completely wanting in coronal tooth structure.

References

1. Kurer, P. F. and Kurer, H. G.: Anchor system for post crown restorations. *Dent Surv,* 45:29–32, Dec. 1969.

2. Standlee, J. P., Caputo, A. A. and Hanson, E. C.: Retention of endodontic dowels: Effects of cement, dowel length, diameter and design. *J Prosthet Dent,* 39:401–405, Apr. 1978.

3. Ruemping, D. R., Lund, M. R. and Schnell, R. J.: Retention of dowels subjected to tensile and torsional forces. *J Prosthet Dent,* 41:159–162, Feb. 1979.

4. Lau, V. S. M.: The reinforcement of endodontically treated teeth. *Dent Clin N Amer,* 20:313–328, Apr. 1976.

5. Perel, M. L. and Muroff, F. I.: Clinical criteria for posts and cores. *J Prosthet Dent,* 28:405–411, Oct. 1972.

6. Sapone, J. and Lorencki, S. F.: An endodontic-prosthodontic approach to internal tooth reinforcement. *J Prosthet Dent,* 45:164–174, Feb. 1981.

7. DiDea, A.: A comparison of two endo-post dowel methods. *Dent Surv,* 47:26, Nov. 1971.

8. Henry, P. J.: Photoelastic analysis of post core restorations. *Aust Dent J,* 22:157–159, Jun. 1977.

9. Standlee, J. P., Caputo, A. A., Collard, E. W. and Pollack, M. H.: Analysis of stress distribution of endodontic posts. *Oral Surg,* 33:952–960, Jun. 1972.

10. Durney, E. C. and Rosen, H.: Root fracture as a complication of post design and insertion: A laboratory study. *Oper Dent,* 2:90–96, Summer 1977.

11. Zmener, O.: Adaptation of threaded dowels to dentin. *J Prosthet Dent,* 43:530–535, May 1980.

12. Kurer, P. F.: Retention of post crowns. A solution of the problem. *Brit Dent J,* 123:167–169, Aug. 1967.

13. Kurer, P. F.: The fin-lock systems for the restoration of endodontically treated teeth. *Brit Dent J,* 148:100–102, Feb. 1980.

14. Kurer, P. F. and Kurer, H. G.: The Kurer Crown Saver. A method of restoration of multi-rooted endodontically treated teeth. *Quint Int,* 8:29–33, Feb. 1977.

15. Stern, N. and Kochavi, D.: Immediate restoration of an endodontically treated tooth by means of a screw-post and composite materials. *Gen Dent,* 25:26–28, Jan. 1977.

16. Kurer, P. F.: The Kurer anchor system for post crown restorations. *J Ont Dent Assoc,* 45:57–60, Feb. 1968.

17. Kurer, H. G., Combe, E. C. and Grant, A. A.: Factors influencing the retention of dowels. *J Prosthet Dent,* 38:515–525, Nov. 1977.

18. Messing, J. J. and Wills, D. J.: Investigation of resistance to stress of screw-threaded crown posts. *J Prosthet Dent,* 30:278–282, Sep. 1973.

Chapter 12

Parallel Self-Threading Dowel

The parallel-sided self-threading dowel* offers a retention device which is intermediate between the stainless steel dowel/composite resin core and the pretapped, parallel threaded crown anchor. The retention afforded by this type of dowel, whose threads are widely separated and shallow, is 94% greater than that for a serrated stainless steel post of the same size. The self-threading anchor is 17% to 45% less retentive than similar sizes of pretapped threaded anchors.[1]

Because the Radix Anchor utilizes threads for much of its retention, it is capable of producing stress in the root. Continuing to thread the anchor after resistance is encountered could result in root fracture or stripping of the threads.[2] If the dowel apex is allowed to engage the supporting tooth structure, high apical stresses will be generated. High stress concentrations will develop in the coronal portion of the root if the coronal flanges of the head come in contact with the root face.[1] In order to avoid these problems, it is recommended that the dowel be reversed or "backed off" a half turn when slight resistance to threading is felt during cementation.

* Radix Anchor System, Star Dental, Syntex Dental Products, Inc., Valley Foege, PA.

TABLE 12-1   **Comparison of Reamer Sizes**

	Diameter (mm.)						
Reamer	1.1	1.2	1.3	1.4	1.5	1.6	1.7
Peeso	No. 3	–	No. 4	–	No. 5	–	No. 6
Maillefer	–	No. 1	–	No. 2	–	–	No. 3

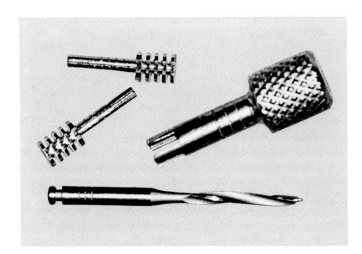

Fig. 12-1   Radix crown anchors are made in three diameters (dowel size exclusive of threads): 1.15 mm., 1.35 mm., and 1.6 mm. The anchors consist of a low profile retentive spiral and a head with five rows of fins or lamellae which retain the composite resin core that is built around it. Maillefer reamers of appropriate matching sizes are used for canal enlargement.

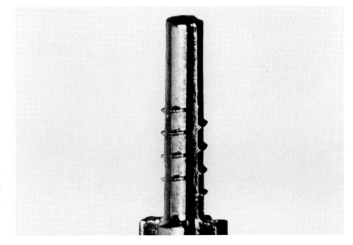

Fig. 12-2 The shallow threaded spiral on the coronal 60% of the dowel is interrupted by four cement vents which run the length of the dowel.

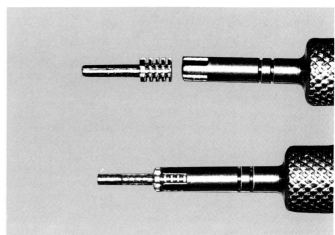

Fig. 12-3 The anchor driver or wrench, used for threading the dowel into the canal, has four prongs (top) which firmly engage four slots in the sides of the head (bottom).

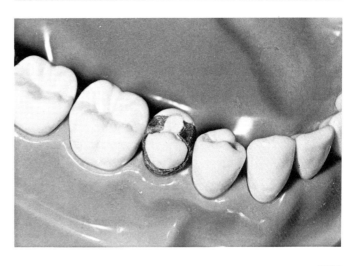

Fig. 12-4 A mandibular premolar in which tooth destruction has been extensive is an ideal indication for the use of the Radix Anchor. Although it can be trimmed for use in other teeth, the anchor works best in teeth whose clinical crowns have some length and volume.

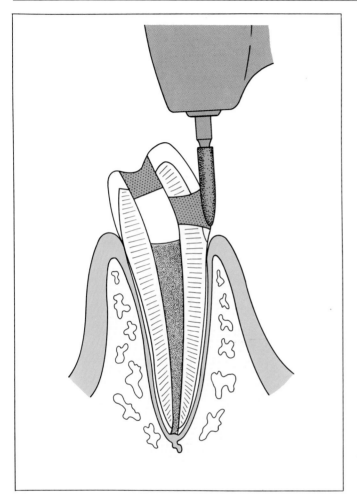

Fig. 12-5 Begin the tooth preparation for the parallel self-threading dowel by removing most of the coronal tooth structure with a diamond in a high speed handpiece.

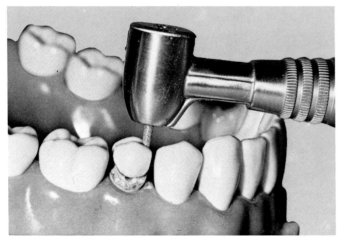

Fig. 12-6 All old restorations are removed as the initial step in this procedure in which it is anticipated that little or no coronal tooth structure will remain. A better assessment of the underlying tooth structure can then be made.

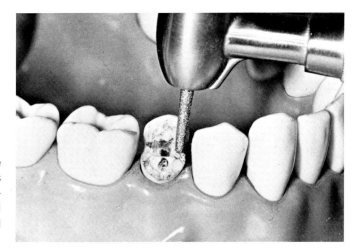

Fig. 12-7 If examination of the coronal tooth structure confirms the initial impression that the clinical crown would be lost, proceed with removing the remaining supragingival tooth structure.

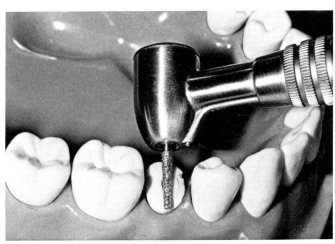

Fig. 12-8 Use the round-end tapered diamond to eliminate the crown by cutting through it at the base. Stay supragingival, if at all possible, and follow the facial-lingual curvature of the interdental papilla.

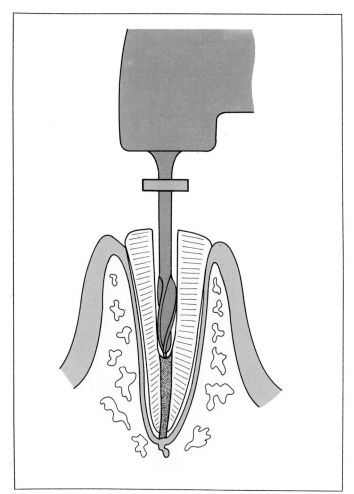

Fig. 12-9   Begin the preparation of the dowel space with Peeso reamers, which are smaller than the matching size Maillefer reamer meant for the chosen size of anchor (see Table 12-1). The reamers are similar in configuration to the Peeso reamers, except for the greater length of the cutting flutes on the Maillefer reamer.

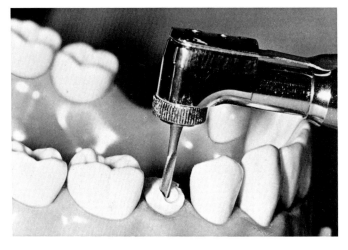

Fig. 12-10   Remove as much gutta percha as possible with a hot endodontic plugger. Choose a landmark or place a rubber stop to gauge the preparation depth. Start with the largest Peeso reamer which will fit in the canal. Then enlarge the canal progressively to the determined width.

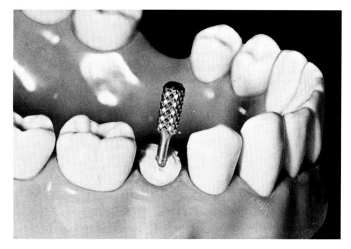

Fig. 12-11 Use the depth gauge in the kit to determine whether adequate depth has been achieved in the dowel space preparation. Insert the gauge into the canal. The mark on the instrument's side should coincide with the edge of the root face.

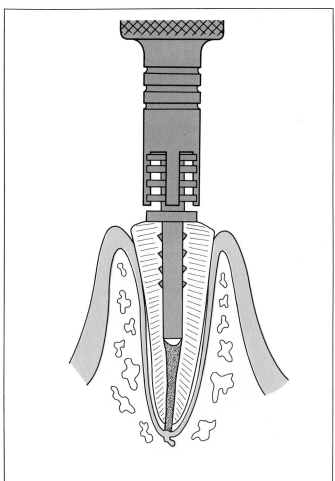

Fig. 12-12 The anchor driver provided with the kit is used initially for tapping the canal and then for reinsertion of the anchor into the tooth during cementation.

281

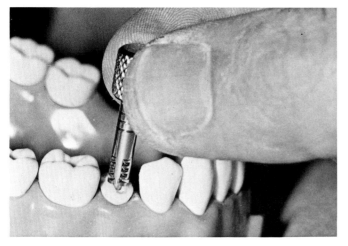

Fig. 12-13 With the driver locked into the head of the anchor, introduce the dowel end into the canal. Use light pressure to tap the walls of the canal. Stop when resistance is encountered. Continuation of the dowel seating after feeling resistance could fracture the root.

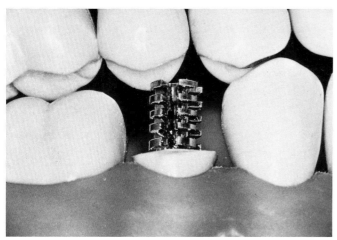

Fig. 12-14 Examine the head when the patient has gently closed. If it is too long, it must be shortened before cementation. If the dowel is short for the size of tooth and crown, shorten the head by cutting off the apical-most row of fins. This will lengthen the dowel at the expense of the head.

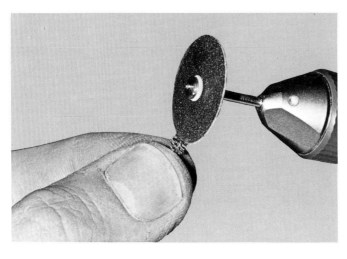

Fig. 12-15 If the head is simply too long occlusally, remove some of the excess length from the top of the head with a 7/8 inch Carborundum separating disc.

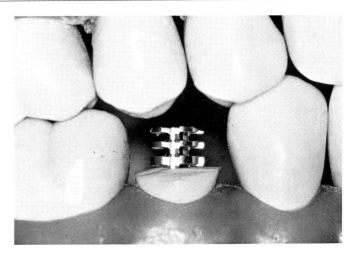

Fig. 12-16　Reseat the dowel and once again check the occlusal clearance on the anchor head. There must be sufficient occlusal clearance to permit the fabrication of a composite resin core and the occlusal surface of the final restoration.

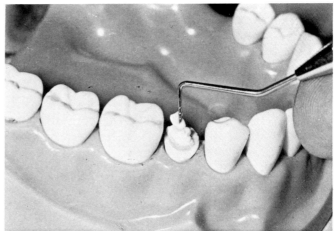

Fig. 12-17　Prepare a thin mix of cement and apply it to the canal with a Lentulo spiral or an endodontic plugger. Coat the walls of the canal liberally with cement.

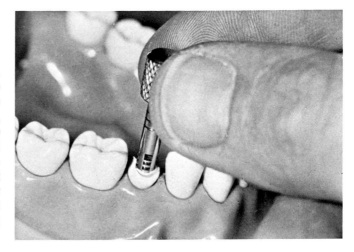

Fig. 12-18　Thread the anchor in, allowing time for the cement to escape along the vents. Stop when resistance is encountered, or permanent damage could be done to the tooth. Best results will be obtained if the anchor is reversed and "backed out" about one-half turn. This insures a low stress dowel without the dowel apex or coronal fins engaging tooth structure.

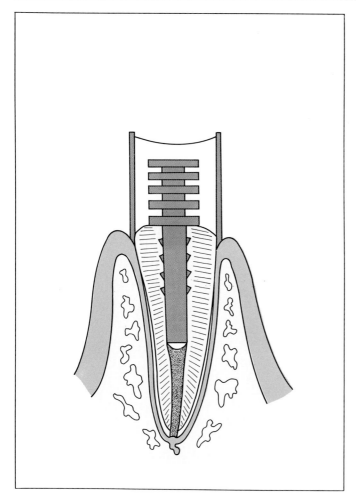

Fig. 12-19 As the cement sets around the dowel, remove the excess from the lamellae of the head and from under the bottommost fin near the root face. The tooth is then ready for fabrication of the composite resin core around the anchor head.

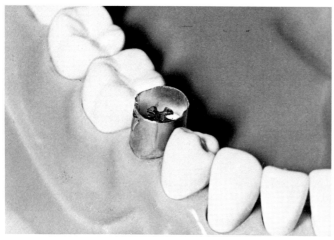

Fig. 12-20 Place a copper band matrix around the tooth being restored. It need not contact the adjacent teeth, since a crown preparation will be made in the composite resin as soon as it has polymerized.

Fig. 12-21 Mix a sizable bulk of opaque composite resin* and load it into the tip of a Centrix syringe.** Green food coloring can be added if a contrast is desired. The conical plunger is inserted into the tip before it is placed in the syringe. Inject the resin around the head of the anchor until the matrix overflows. Place a fingertip over the band to compress the composite resin around the lamellae.

* Concise Crown Build-up Material, 3-M Dental Products, St. Paul, MN.
** Centrix C-R Syringe, Centrix Inc., Stratford, CT.

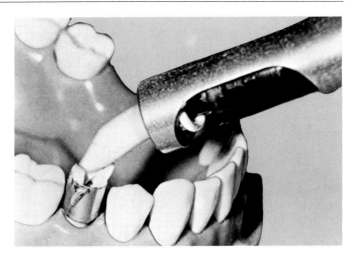

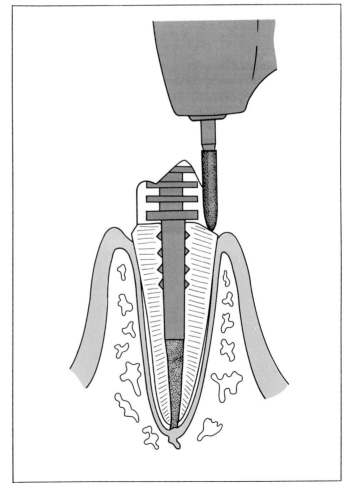

Fig. 12-22 The preparation for the final restoration will be made in the composite resin core with a diamond stone in a high speed handpiece.

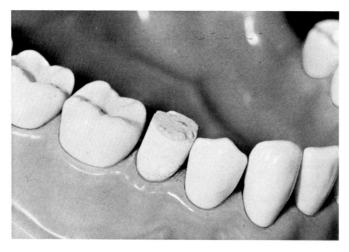

Fig. 12-23 The composite resin surrounding the anchor head forms a blank from which the crown preparation can be shaped.

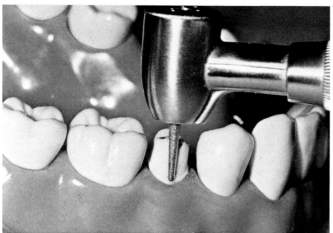

Fig. 12-24 Generous occlusal and axial reduction are accomplished with a round-end tapered diamond. Do not be concerned if portions of the fins are exposed during the preparation. The crown preparation finish line must be placed considerably apical to the margin of the composite resin to minimize any possibility of leakage.[3]

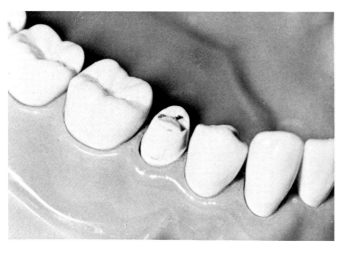

Fig. 12-25 The completed preparation which has been made largely in the composite resin core has the configuration of an ideal porcelain fused to metal crown preparation. Occlusal clearance should be a minimum of 1.5 mm.

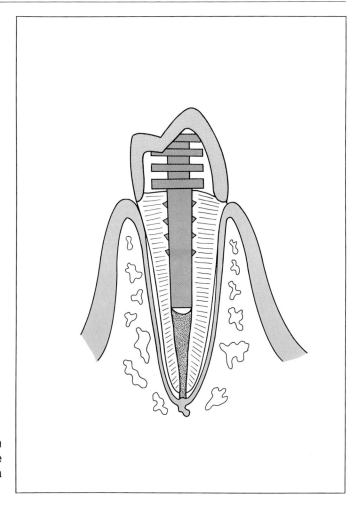

Fig. 12-26 The final restoration is placed over the composite resin core which is retained with a Radix Anchor.

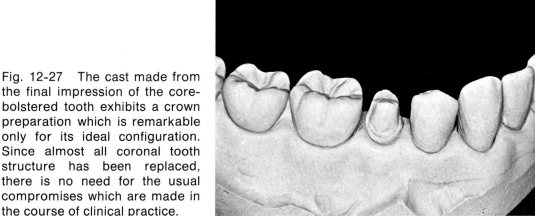

Fig. 12-27 The cast made from the final impression of the core-bolstered tooth exhibits a crown preparation which is remarkable only for its ideal configuration. Since almost all coronal tooth structure has been replaced, there is no need for the usual compromises which are made in the course of clinical practice.

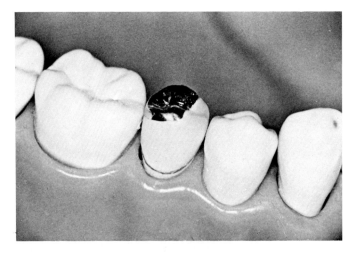

Fig. 12-28 The completed porcelain fused to metal crown employed to restore a broken down premolar with no good coronal tooth structure.

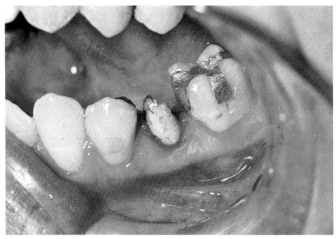

Fig. 12-29 Following endodontic treatment, there was virtually no sound coronal tooth structure remaining. The unsupported tooth structure was eliminated with a diamond.

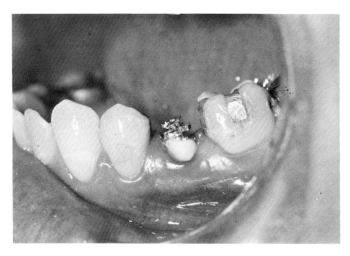

Fig. 12-30 The Radix Anchor was cemented in place to provide retention for the composite resin core. In order to provide sufficient occlusal clearance for the core, only two rows of lamellae are left on the anchor head. Three were removed *before* the anchor was cemented.

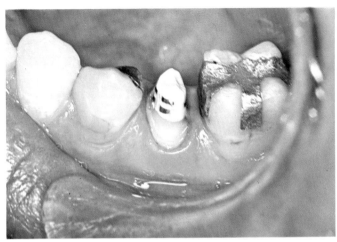

Fig. 12-31 After the composite resin core is added around the head, a crown preparation is made on the tooth. Tooth, resin, and metal head have been cut to produce the occlusal and axial configuration of a crown preparation.

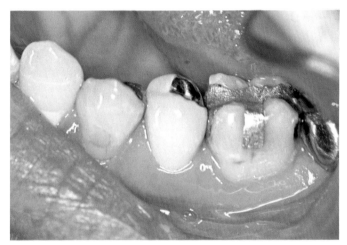

Figure 12-32 The completed crown provides a suitable restoration of this tooth whose restoration without a dowel-core would have produced a result with a doubtful prognosis.

References

1. Standlee, J. P., Caputo, A. A., Holcomb, J. and Trabert, K. C.: The retentive and stress-distributing properties of a threaded endodontic dowel. *J Prosthet Dent,* 44:398–404, Oct. 1980.

2. Spang, H.: The Radix-Anchor system (II)–the reconstruction of severely eroded single-rooted teeth. *Quint Int,* 6:55–62, Oct. 1975.

3. Eissmann, H. F. and Radke, R. A.: Post-endodontic restoration. In Cohen, S. and Burns, R. C.: *Pathways of the Pulp,* St. Louis, C. V. Mosby Co., 1976, p. 550.

Chapter 13

Tapered Self-Threading Dowel

This style of dowel has been in use for over 50 years.[1] It is the simplest of all the threaded dowels. The taper of the dowels is variable. Many of them have two tapers: one at the tip and another for the main body of the thread. The taper for the tip can be as little as 10° and as much as 30°, being less on long, thin dowels and greater on short, thick ones. The taper on the main body of the thread can range from 0° (parallel-sided) to 3.0°. The use of this type of dowel is the prime example of the use of the root canal as the "ultimate pin hole." An amalgam or composite resin core is usually fabricated around the dowel after it is cemented.

Because of its dowel size and the bulky head, tapered self-threading dowels are generally restricted to use in molars. The large size of the dowel head (2.6 mm. long and 1.6 mm. across) and the relatively small circumference of an anterior tooth do not allow an adequate bulk of core material in most cases.[2] It is frequently used on teeth with a minimum of coronal tooth structure and multiple divergent canals. The non-parallel relationship adds to the retentive qualities of the self-threaded dowel.[3] Its use should be reserved primarily for single tooth restorations.

The tapered self-threading dowel is simple and easy to use. The fact that it engages dentin with its threads unquestionably provides excellent retention. Its most obvious advantage is that the dowel-core can be placed in a single appointment. Often this can be the appointment during which the endodontic obturation is accomplished. In this case, isolation of the tooth can be maintained throughout the procedure, making the dowel more an extension of the endodontic filling than a separate restorative procedure.

However, this type of dowel also produces high stress concentrations,[4] with its wedge-like action producing stress concentrations more severe than those seen in other types of threaded dowels.[5] Translated into practical terms, this means that there is a danger of cracking a root.[6] The danger of root fracture is most acute when excessive torque is applied,[7] or when the dowel is over-twisted.[2] Torque required to seat the dowel increases with diameter, but dowel length seems to exert no influence.[7] Larger diameter dowels have been observed to cause root fractures, especially in teeth with ovoid canals.[8] Dowels which are oversized for their prepared canal also represent a hazard to the tooth. A dowel that is too large compresses dentin and increases the risk of root fracture.[3]

Durney and Rosen found that the torque required to insert a tapered, self-threading dowel was approximately one-fourth of the torque needed to fracture a root experimentally.[7] They suggest that these dowels should be turned slowly and delicately without leverage. This would seem to be an adequate safety margin, but clinically it has not always proven to be so. It may simply be that this type of dowel has been used in too many poorly selected weak roots by careless operators. Whatever the cause, the recommendation has been made that tapered, self-threading dowels be passively cemented in slightly oversized canals.[9, 10] In a slight modification of that technique, Tidmarsh has suggested that a dowel with a "snug, sliding fit" be cemented, engaging the threads no more than a single turn during seating.[11]

Tapered self-threading dowels have been implicated in corrosion which could result in root fracture.[12] Rud and Omnell examined 468 teeth with vertical or oblique root fractures and concluded that 72% of the fractures resulted from corrosion.[13] It was theorized that galvanic reactions caused the formation of corrosive products that fractured the teeth.[14] It is also possible that the teeth were fractured at the time of insertion, or subsequently, with the fracture remaining undetected for a period of time. The fracture, however minute, would permit the free passage of saliva and/or serum into contact with the dowel and crown, causing corrosion products to be formed *after* the fracture.

Nonetheless, it is recommended that the dowel be examined prior to insertion. Confirm that the electroplated gold surface is still intact, protecting the brass body which is 60% copper and 40% zinc. Further, that portion of the dowel to be placed in the canal should not be cut or prepared. Derand recommends that the core be placed during the same appointment at which the dowel is cemented.[12] This will prevent the cement around the dowel from being exposed to the fluids of the oral cavity for any prolonged period.

Tapered self-threading dowels have been marketed under a number of different brands, with small differences in instrumentation or packaging. The Dentatus Screw Post* is the most commonly used of this style of dowel. Currently, it is marketed in a stainless steel and a gold-plated brass dowel.

* Dentatus Screw Post, Union Broach Corp., Long Island City, NY.

Fig. 13-1 Dentatus Screw Posts are available in six diameters: 1.0 mm., 1.2 mm., 1.3 mm., 1.5 mm., 1.6 mm., and 1.8 mm. Although corresponding size engine reamers are available, the technique described in this chapter is accomplished with Peeso reamers. There are four lengths of dowels: 7.8 mm., 9.3 mm., 11.8 mm., and 14.2 mm. The head of each screw post is square, with two crossing slots on the end. There are two seating wrenches provided with the system.

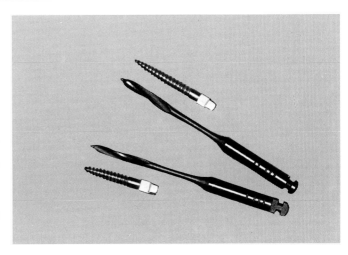

Fig. 13-2 One wrench is designed to fit internally into the head of the dowel to allow placement of the dowel in tight areas. It also permits insertion of a dowel whose head shape and size have been altered. If the brass dowels are used, the metal head can be easily reduced, if necessary.

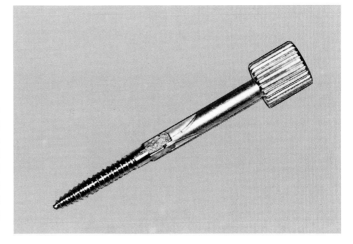

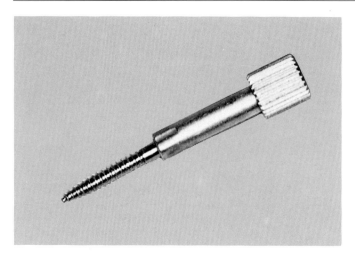

Fig. 13-3 A second wrench fits over the head of the dowel. It is useful on severely broken-down teeth in which the dowel head is unaltered.

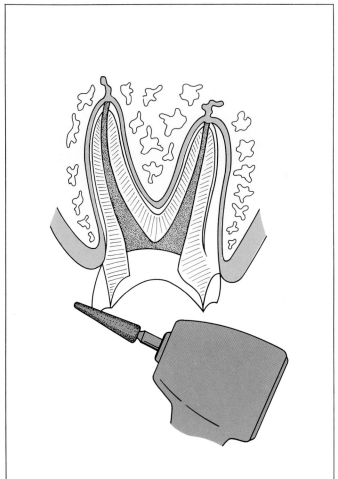

Fig. 13-4 The Dentatus Screw Post should be considered for molar teeth in which the restoration of the coronal portion of the tooth is beyond the scope of the typical pin-retained core. The decision on the best technique for restoring a given tooth should be reserved until all restorations and unsupported tooth structure have been removed.

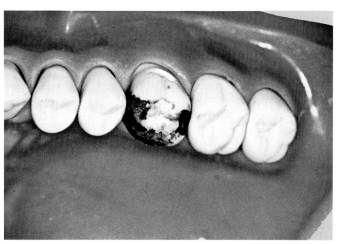

Fig. 13-5 A typical situation that may be suited for a restoration using the tapered self-threading dowel is an endodontically treated molar with a large existing amalgam and carious involvement of remaining tooth structure.

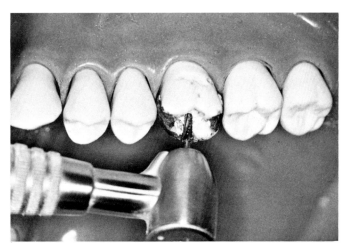

Fig. 13-6 The initial step in the restoration of such a tooth is the removal of all cements, existing restorations, and bases.

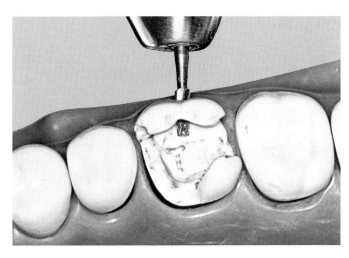

Fig. 13-7 Any caries are excavated, and questionable or unsupported tooth structure is removed.

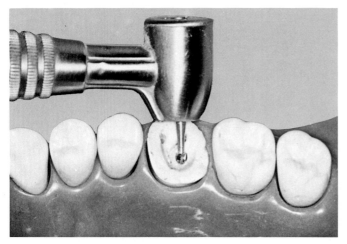

Fig. 13-8 At this point, the tooth is evaluated. What is the best means of restoring the missing coronal tooth structure? Consideration should be given to the functional demands on the tooth, i.e., single tooth restoration, bridge abutment, or removable partial denture abutment. Another important factor is the amount of intact clinical crown. In this case there is insufficient bulk of tooth structure around the root canals for placement of pins or other retentive features.

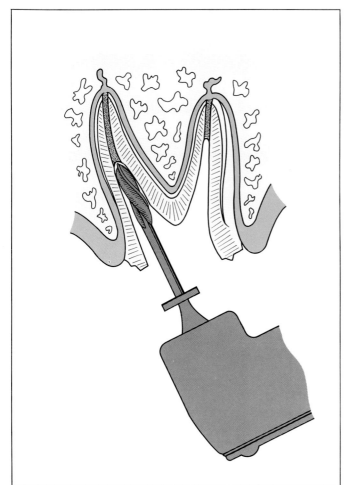

Fig. 13-9 The dowel spaces are now prepared in the straightest and bulkiest roots. In most cases, it is possible to place two dowels. The distal canal of a mandibular molar and the palatal canal of a maxillary molar are usually the best suited to accommodate the primary dowel.

Fig. 13-10 Length and diameter are determined for the dowel. It should be as long as possible, but not closer than 4.0 mm. from the apex. Length often will be limited by root curvature. A Peeso reamer is chosen that will fit into the canal easily. Gutta percha is removed with a hot instrument, and the space is enlarged with a series of reamers until the desired diameter is reached. A comparison of the diameters of Peeso reamers and Dentatus Screw Posts is shown in Table 13-1.

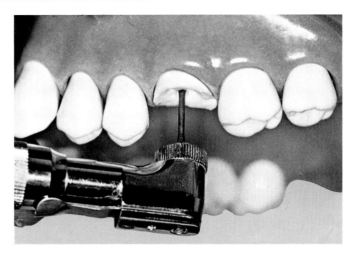

TABLE 13-1 **Comparison of Reamer and Dowel Sizes**

	Diameter (mm.)									
	0.9	1.0	1.1	1.2	1.3	1.4	1.5	1.6	1.7	1.8
Peeso Reamer	No. 2	–	No. 3	–	No. 4	–	No. 5	–	No. 6	–
Dentatus Screw Post	–	No. 1	–	No. 2	No. 3	–	No. 4	No. 5	–	No. 6

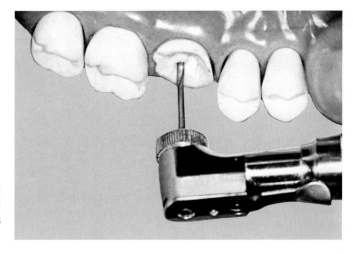

Fig. 13-11 The second dowel space is prepared. The distofacial canal has been selected on this maxillary first molar.

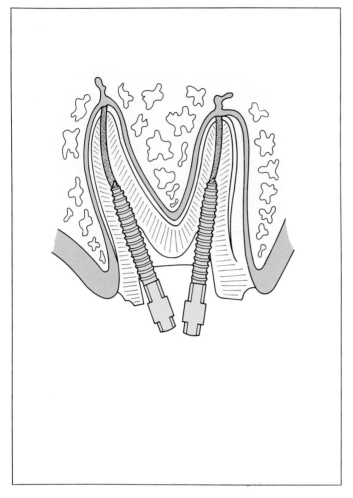

Fig. 13-12 The Dentatus Screw Posts are prepared for cementation by trying them in and making any necessary adjustments.

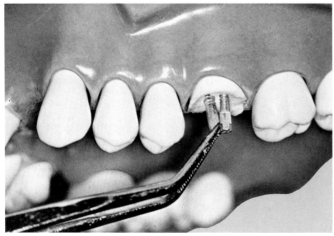

Fig. 13-13 Place the dowels into the canals. They should slide freely to within 0.5–1.0 mm. of the depths of their prepared spaces. The additional length will be gained when each dowel is locked into the dentin. The dowels must be tried in together to determine whether the heads need to be reduced or reshaped to allow both dowels to be seated.

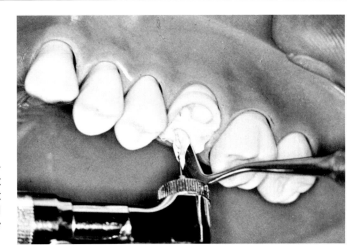

Fig. 13-14 Either polycarboxylate or zinc phosphate cement can be used. Place the cement into the canal with a Lentulo spiral and coat each dowel generously with cement.

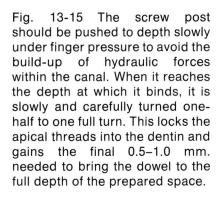

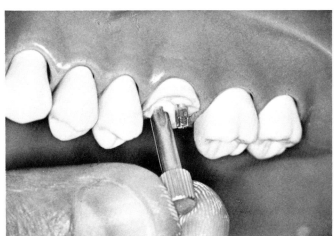

Fig. 13-15 The screw post should be pushed to depth slowly under finger pressure to avoid the build-up of hydraulic forces within the canal. When it reaches the depth at which it binds, it is slowly and carefully turned one-half to one full turn. This locks the apical threads into the dentin and gains the final 0.5–1.0 mm. needed to bring the dowel to the full depth of the prepared space.

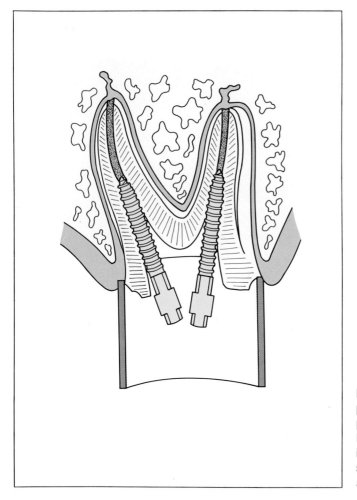

Fig. 13-16 An amalgam or composite resin core can now be placed. No auxiliary pins will be needed, unless only one dowel is used. In such cases, pins should be placed as anti-rotational retentive components.

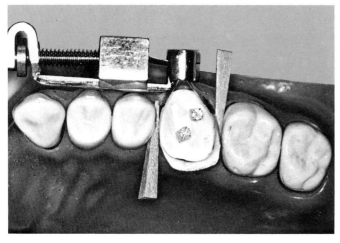

Fig. 13-17 The dowel head should not be too close to the outer perimeter of the projected axial contours of the prepared core. Neither should they be closer than 2.0–2.5 mm. from the opposing occlusion. If necessary, they should be altered. The space between the two heads should also allow a bulk of core material. A matrix band is placed and the core material of choice is inserted. If possible, wedges should be used to minimize gingival flash.

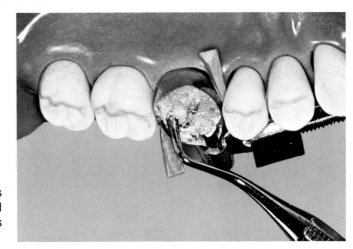

Fig. 13-18 Amalgam cores should be carefully condensed into the chamber area, as well as around each dowel.

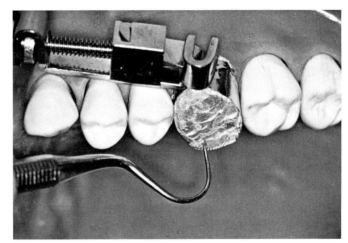

Fig. 13-19 Excess amalgam is removed while the matrix band is still in place.

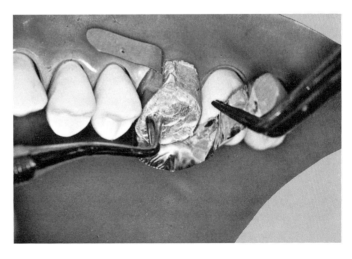

Fig. 13-20 As soon as the initial set has begun, the matrix can be removed. A large condenser is held on the occlusal surface of the soft amalgam to prevent dislodging it during removal of the matrix.

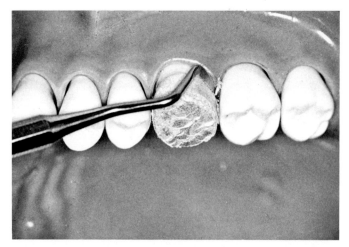

Fig. 13-21 At this point, all gingival flash is removed. This allows for the core to exist in a healthy state for some time, if needed. Exposing the gingival margin now will make finish line preparation that much easier at a later time.

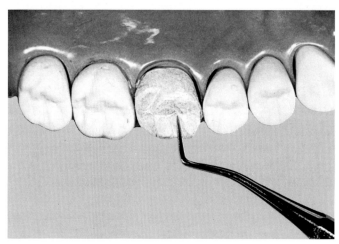

Fig. 13-22 The final preparation can be roughed out by carving the soft amalgam. If the core is scheduled for final preparation in the near future, the interproximal contacts can be carved away at this time. This will make preparation of these areas much easier.

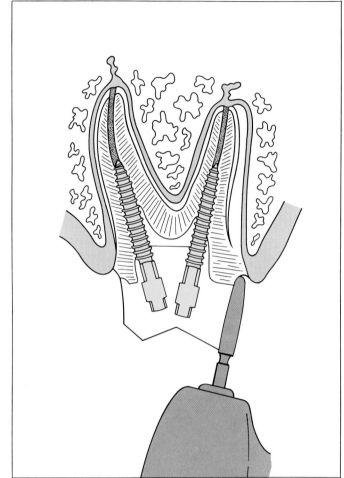

Fig. 13-23 Preparation of the core is accomplished with burs and diamonds as though it were tooth structure. On an amalgam core of this size, preparation is probably best delayed until a subsequent appointment. Use of a spherical high copper amalgam* will achieve a hard enough set to do the preparation at the same appointment. Even its surface is more easily instrumented at a later appointment, however.

* Tytin, S.S. White Dental Products Int'l., Philadelphia, PA.

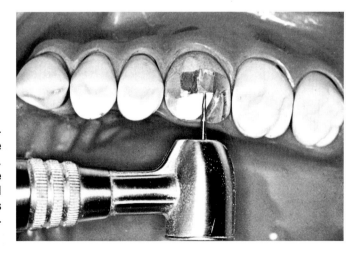

Fig. 13-24 The occlusal reduction already carved into the amalgam is refined, using a No. 170 nondentate fissure bur. If the dowel is accidentally exposed during the crown preparation, it is easily cut and results in no excessive vibration.

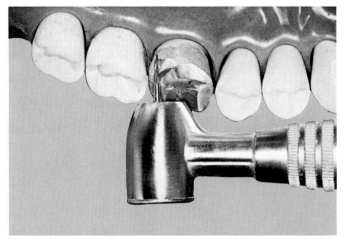

Fig. 13-25 The functional cusp bevel is placed with the same instrument. The occlusal reduction is evaluated at this time. For a porcelain fused to metal crown preparation, it should be a minimum of 1.5 mm. for the entire occlusal surface.

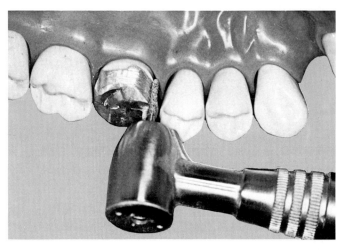

Fig. 13-26 Begin the lingual axial reduction, using a chamfer diamond. Be sure that the finish line is apical to the margin of the amalgam core. The crown finish line should be placed on solid tooth structure.

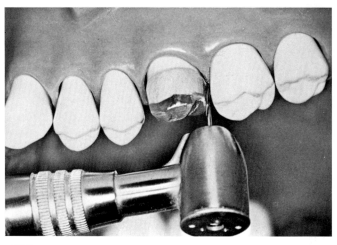

Fig. 13-27 The initial interproximal cuts are made with a small diameter, tapered fissure bur, such as a No. 169 L.

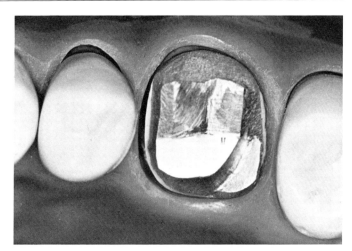

Fig. 13-28 The narrow shoulder or ledge formed by this bur will allow visualization of the finish line interproximally. Any amalgam seen on this shoulder should be removed.

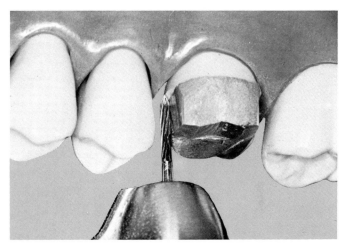

Fig. 13-29 When the shoulder is apical to amalgam, a bevel can be placed on it, essentially converting it to a chamfer. If a chamfer had been placed initially, it would have been difficult to confirm that the finish line was on tooth structure rather than on amalgam.

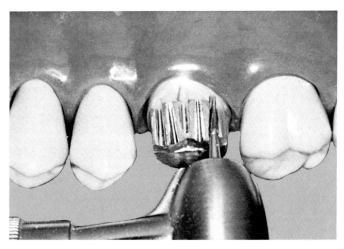

Fig. 13-30 Place depth orientation grooves to a depth of 1.5 mm. on the facial axial surface with the No. 170 bur.

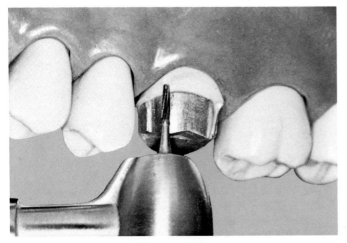

Fig. 13-31 Complete facial axial reduction, removing the tooth structure between the depth grooves. A shoulder finish line is instrumented to allow for an adequate bulk of metal and porcelain.

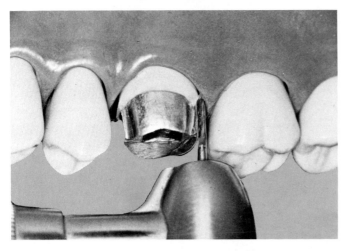

Fig. 13-32 A bevel is placed on the shoulder and blended into the interproximal chamfers.

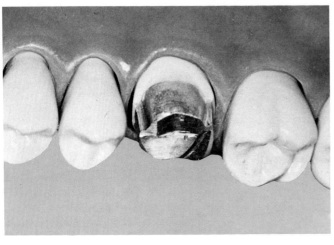

Fig. 13-33 The completed porcelain fused to metal preparation is seen in an amalgam core retained by Dentatus Screw Posts.

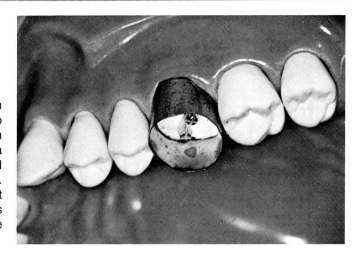

Fig. 13-34 A composite resin core may also be utilized to replace the missing coronal tooth structure. A copper band or a celluloid core form can be used when constructing a resin core. Since this core will be prepared at the same appointment, contours and interproximal contacts are not a concern.

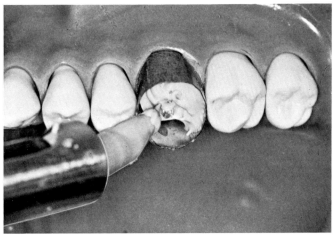

Fig. 13-35 The composite resin* is placed with a Centrex syringe.** Enlarge the hole in the tip to allow easy injection of the bulk of material needed for a core. The material can be colored with green food coloring to facilitate differentiation from tooth structure in a deep sulcus.

* Concise Crown Build-up Material, 3-M Dental Products, St. Paul, MN
** Centrix C-R Syringe, Centrix Inc., Stratford, CT.

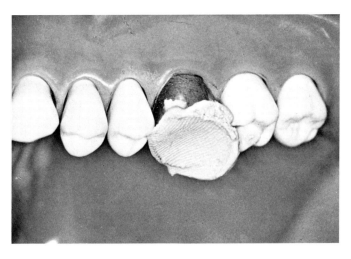

Fig. 13-36 When the copper band is full, place a finger firmly over the top and hold it until the material has set. This produces a bulky composite resin core with a fingerprint on the occlusal surface.

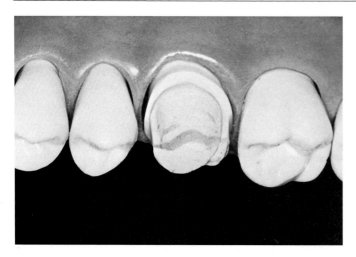

Fig. 13-37 The crown preparation for the porcelain fused to metal restoration is completed in composite resin as it was in amalgam.

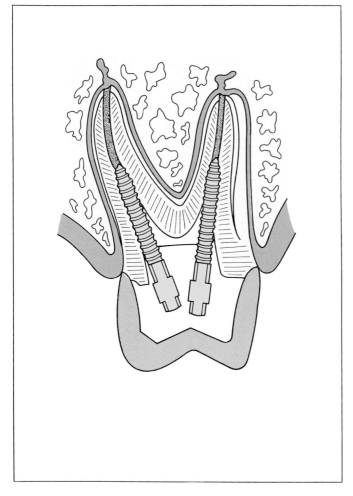

Fig. 13-38 The crown can be fabricated over the core in the usual manner.

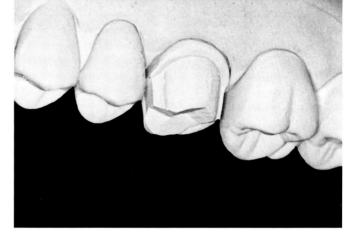

Fig. 13-39 An impression is made and the cast is poured. On the cast, the prepared tooth is identical to a preparation in natural tooth structure except that it is usually a more nearly ideal preparation.

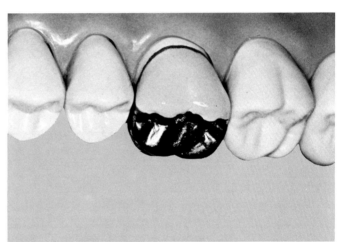

Fig. 13-40 The completed porcelain fused to metal restoration.

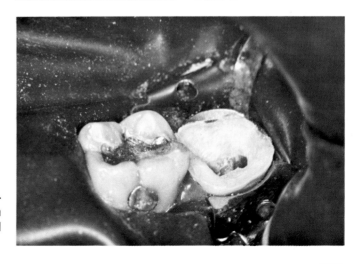

Fig. 13-41 This mandibular second molar was severely broken down, with no remaining coronal tooth structure.

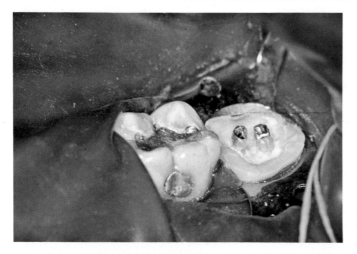

Fig. 13-42 The Dentatus Screw Posts were cemented, and the large heads were reshaped to allow for an adequate bulk of core material.

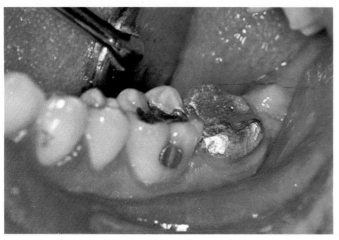

Fig. 13-43 The amalgam core is shown after condensation and rough carving.

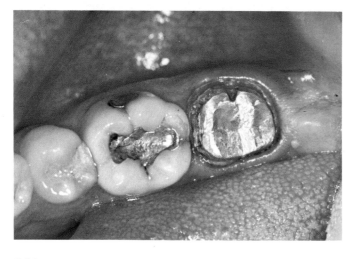

Fig. 13-44 Final preparation of the core is completed with all finish lines on solid tooth structure.

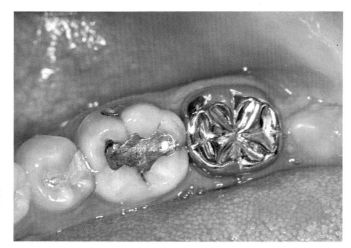

Fig. 13-45 A full veneer gold crown completes the restoration of a crownless non-vital tooth that would have been extremely difficult to replace satisfactorily with a prosthetic device.

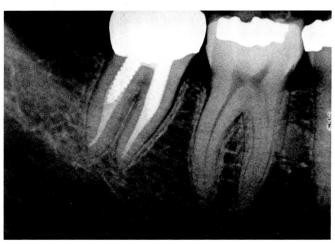

Fig. 13-46 A radiograph shows the tapered self-threading dowels of acceptable lengths with adequate gutta percha to form a predictable apical seal.

References

1. Le Gro, A. L.: *Ceramics in Dentistry,* Brooklyn, Dental Items of Interest Publishing Co., 1925, p. 58.

2. Herschman, J. B., Weine, F. S. and Strauss, S.: Restoration of the endodontically treated tooth. In Weine, F. S.: *Endodontic Therapy.* St. Louis: C. V. Mosby Co., 1976, pp. 444–475.

3. Johnson, J. K., Schwartz, N. L. and Blackwell, R. T.: Evaluation and restoration of endodontically treated posterior teeth. *JADA,* 93:597–605, Sep. 1976.

4. Henry, P. J.: Photoelastic analysis of post core restorations. *Aust Dent J,* 22:157–159, Jun. 1977.

5. Standlee, J. P., Caputo, A. A. and Holcomb, J.: The Dentatus Screw: Comparative stress analysis with other endodontic dowel designs. *J Oral Rehab.* In press.

6. Perel, M. L. and Muroff, F. I.: Clinical criteria for posts and cores. *J Prosthet Dent,* 28:405–411, Oct. 1972.

7. Durney, E. C. and Rosen, H.: Root fracture as a complication of post design and insertion: A laboratory study. *Oper Dent,* 2:90–96, Summer 1977.

8. Zmener, O.: Adaptation of threaded dowels to dentin. *J Prosthet Dent,* 43:530–535, May 1980.

9. Caputo, A. A. and Standlee, J. P.: Pins and posts–why, when, and how. *Dent Clin N Amer,* 20:299–311, Apr. 1976.

10. Goerig, A. C. and Mueninghoff, L. A.: Management of the endodontically treated tooth. Part I. Philosophy for restoration design. *J Prosthet Dent.* In press.

11. Tidmarsh, B.: Restoration of endodontically treated posterior teeth. *J Endo,* 2:374–375, Dec. 1976.

12. Derand, T.: Corrosion of screwposts. *Odont Revy,* 22:371–378, 1971.

13. Rud, J. and Omnell, K. A.: Root fractures due to corrosion. Diagnostic aspects. *Scand J Dent Res,* 78:397–403, 1970.

14. Angmar-Mansson, B., Omnell, K. A. and Rud, J.: Root fractures due to corrosion. I. Metallurgical aspects. *Odont Revy,* 20:244–265, 1969.

Chapter 14

Amalgam Pin Core

Not every endodontically treated tooth will require the use of a dowel in its canal to retain the core and assist the crown in withstanding occlusal forces. Most molars, in fact, can be successfully restored without a dowel. Their greater circumference generally eliminates the necessity of a dowel to bolster the tooth.[1]

Amalgam has been popular for this purpose because of its availability, ease of manipulation, strength, and familiarity. Pins were described for anchoring amalgam in teeth with extensive coronal damage over thirty years ago by Markley.[2] It was not long before pin-retained amalgam was presented as a foundation for cast restorations in badly broken-down teeth.[3] Although amalgam pin cores have been widely used for molars, they are not usually employed in the restoration of premolars and anterior teeth. These teeth lack the bulk of tooth structure between the pulp chamber and the outside of the tooth to hold pins securely and still keep them embedded in amalgam when the core is reduced for placement of the final crown.

Pins were thought at one time to reinforce the amalgam, but Wing,[4] Going,[5] Welk and Dilts[6] found the amalgam to be weakened by the presence of pins. They are placed to aid in the retention of the core and not to strengthen it.[7]

The retention of the amalgam core is subject to several variables. Depth of insertion of the pins into dentin will play a role in their retention. The optimum depth for self-threading pins has been put at 2.0 mm.,[8] while the depth of cemented pins is 3-4 mm.[9] The pin should also extend 2.0 mm. from the tooth into the amalgam.[8]

Self-threading pins are the most retentive of all pins. Dilts and associates found them to be approximately five times as retentive as cemented pins,[9] and Moffa et al. reported a similar superiority.[8] Although self-threading pins do provide excellent retention, there are some reservations about their use in endodontically treated teeth[10] because they have been shown to produce crazing during insertion.[11, 12] Placing the pin holes at least 0.5 mm. from the dentino-enamel junction decreases the chances for crazing, as does the use of 0.6 mm. pins instead of 0.8 mm. pins.[11] The use of sharp drills also helps to minimize the production of dentinal defects.[12]

In spite of the possibility of fracturing tooth structure, self-threading pins are seen as an acceptable risk. They provide superior retention, and they do not have to be embedded as deeply in dentin.[13]

When cores fail, it seems to happen between the pin and tooth structure. Adaptation of amalgam to retentive pins is excellent microscopically, which would suggest good retention of amalgam to the pins.[14] This is, in fact, borne out experimentally by Fujimoto et al., who found that amalgam's separating from pins accounted for only 4.2% of core failures.[15] Fractures of dentin accounted for most failures of amalgam cores in that study, and the incidence of that mode of failure increased as the number of pins exceeded three.

This is generally consistent with the empirical recommendation of one pin for each missing line angle of tooth structure,[16] one pin per missing cusp,[17] and one pin per missing wall.[10, 18] While these recommendations fall short of the urge to ring the tooth with a forest of pins, they take into account the fact that as the number of pins is increased to produce greater retention, the amalgam and dentin are simultaneously weakened.

Alternative proposals have been made for the retention of an amalgam core. Gold platinum dowels[19] and 0.9 mm. orthodontic wire[20] have been inserted in the canal as a modified form of dowel-core. A retention slot around the periphery of a crownless tooth has been described by Outhwaite et al.[21] The slot, which is the width and depth of a No. 33½ bur, retained cores as well as four self-threading pins. Nayyar and associates employ a coronal-radicular amalgam dowel-core which fills the pulp chamber and 2-4 mm. of each canal of a molar with amalgam.[22] The bulk of amalgam is utilized for both strength and retention.

Since composite resin cores can be placed more quickly and easily than amalgam cores, why is amalgam still used? Laboratory studies indicate similar tensile strength when the two materials are employed in cores.[15] Crowns cemented to amalgam cores are significantly more retentive initially than those cemented to composite resin cores, although the composite resin cores gain retentive strength with the passage of time.[23]

Amalgam has been used quite successfully for a number of years. It is a known quantity. Composite resin restorations utilized in other applications have a record of being less durable. Crowns which are placed over amalgam or composite resin cores exhibit significantly greater microleakage than crowns placed over preparations in natural tooth structure.[24] When this is coupled with the fact that composite resin cores show significantly more leakage than amalgam cores,[25] there is a potential for leakage into the canal and subsequent endodontic failure. Every practitioner must weigh these factors in selecting a core material and technique.

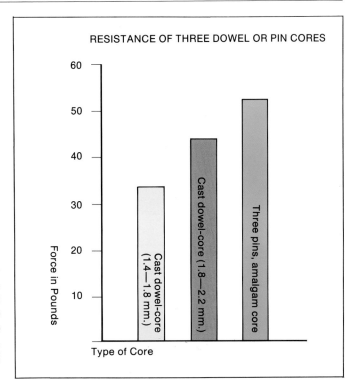

Fig. 14-1 In a study of resistance to obliquely directed forces, amalgam cores retained by three 0.6 mm. self-threading pins were significantly more difficult to displace than cast dowel-cores. (Based on data by Lovdahl and Nichols.[26])

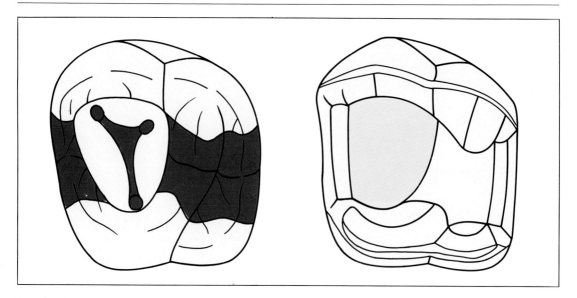

Fig. 14-2   An important aspect of restoring endodontically treated posterior teeth is knowing when to use amalgam pin cores and when to resort to some form of dowel-core. When destruction of tooth structure is limited to a moderate M.O.D. restoration, plus the endodontic access, it is possible to restore the tooth properly by using an M.O.D. onlay.

Fig. 14-3   If one cusp has been destroyed in addition to the tooth preparation required for a minimal M.O.D. restoration, a full veneer crown without an amalgam core can be used. A pin may be required in the casting. If the destruction of tooth structure is more than minimal, an amalgam core may be desirable, although it could be placed without pins, extending into the pulp chamber as described by Nayyar.[22]

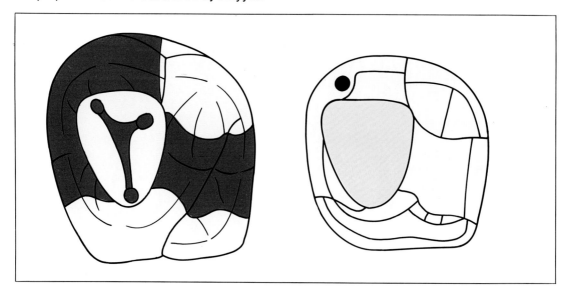

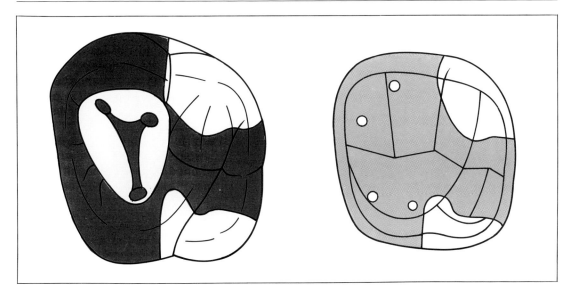

Fig. 14-4 When two cusps have been destroyed, an amalgam pin core is indicated, with one or two pins in each cusp area. The supragingival tooth structure remaining in the two cusps is a necessary part of the retention and resistance of the amalgam core.

Fig. 14-5 If only one cusp of coronal tooth structure is remaining, it is possible to use an amalgam pin core. If the intact cusp is a bulky one, three pins will probably suffice.

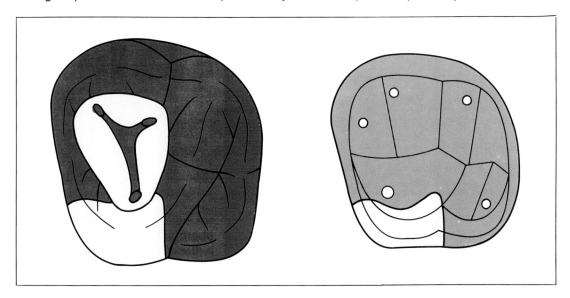

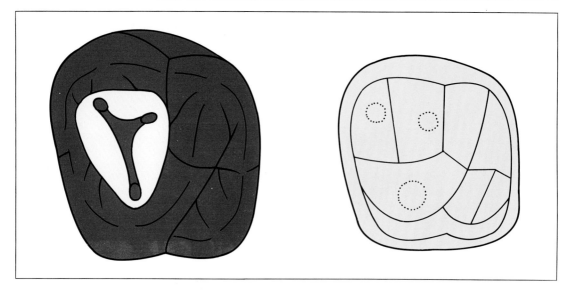

Fig. 14-6   A molar which has lost all of its coronal tooth structure is a poor risk for a simple amalgam pin core. It no longer has the remaining coronal tooth structure needed for additional retention of the core.[13] The use of dowels can provide some resistance to horizontally directed forces. If the tooth is being restored as a single crown, stainless steel dowels or passively fitting self-threading dowels can be used with an amalgam core. However, if the molar is to serve as a fixed bridge abutment, it should be built up with a two-piece cast dowel-core.

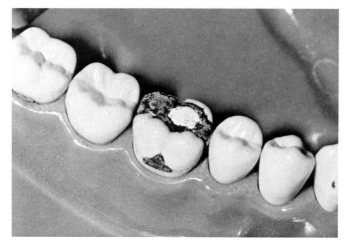

Fig. 14-7   An extensively damaged molar with at least two sound cusps is an excellent candidate for an amalgam pin core build-up.

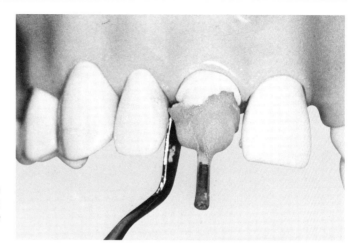

Fig. 14-8 A lingual view of the tooth shows typically weakened lingual cusps. One has already fractured.

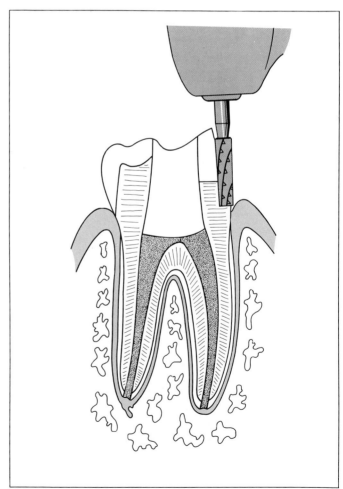

Fig. 14-9 When the use of an amalgam pin core is anticipated, previous restorations, bases and caries are removed first.

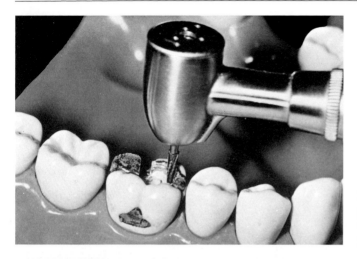

Fig. 14-10 The large, old amalgam restoration can be removed with a diamond, an amalgam bur, or a large crosscut fissure bur.

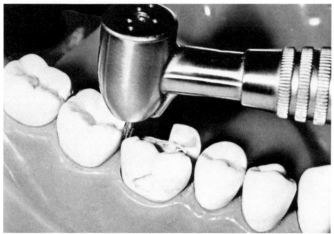

Fig. 14-11 *All* of the old amalgam is removed, including small separate axial restorations such as the Class V amalgam shown here. Only then is it possible to make an accurate assessment of the quantity and quality of remaining tooth structure.

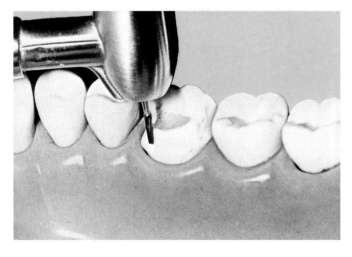

Fig. 14-12 Peripheral areas are shaped to produce maximum retention and resistance. Because lingual cusps were missing or badly undermined, a wide gingival shoulder extends all the way around the lingual surface, tying in with the gingival floor of both the mesial and distal boxes.

Fig. 14-13 Pin holes are placed with a twist drill in areas of bulk. While pin location is an important part of an amalgam pin core, it is not as critical on the endodontically treated tooth as it is on the vital tooth.

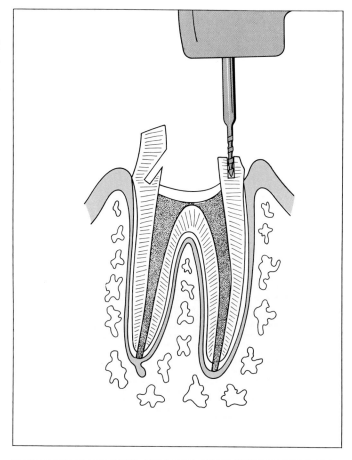

Fig. 14-14 Pin placement should favor the dentino-enamel junction by being close to the pulp chamber.[13] This permits the pin to be in a bulk of dentin, to minimize crazing and avoid lateral perforation. Primary sites for pins are on the mesial and distal surfaces near line angles. Secondary locations can be used if primary sites are unusable. Interproximal surfaces with concavities and areas overlying furcations are unacceptable because of the risk of lateral perforation. (After Fisher.)

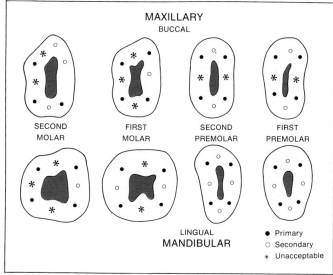

MAXILLARY
BUCCAL

SECOND MOLAR

FIRST MOLAR

SECOND PREMOLAR

FIRST PREMOLAR

LINGUAL
MANDIBULAR

● Primary
○ Secondary
✻ Unacceptable

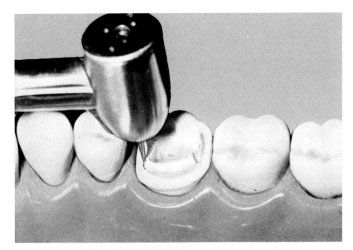

Fig. 14-15 Start all pin holes with a No. ½ round bur, which allows precise placement of the channel. If the hole is started with a drill, there is a great risk of its skipping or slipping.[27]

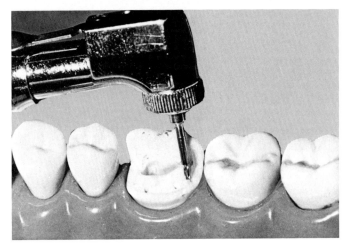

Fig. 14-16 The pin hole should be made with quick, forceful thrusts. Use a minimum number of insertions to drill the pin hole.[17, 28] Repeated withdrawals and reinsertions overenlarge the channel and increase the risk of twist drill fracture. Keep track of the number of pin holes cut by any one drill. Do not attempt to place any more than 20 pin holes with one instrument.[12]

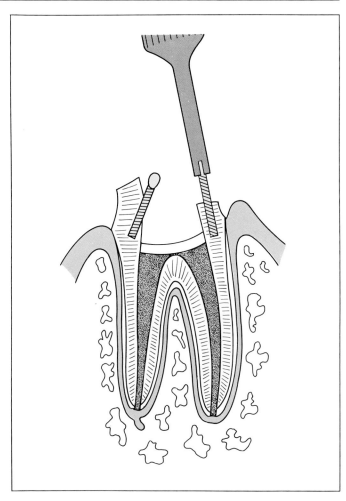

Fig. 14-17 Insert pins into their holes. Avoid overtorquing the pins because this produces stress and can lead to crazing of the dentin.

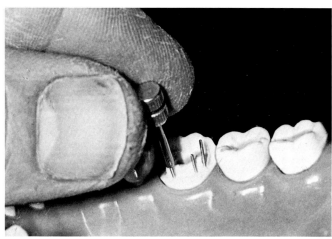

Fig. 14-18 A hand wrench affords a proprioceptive safeguard against overseating the pins if a light touch is employed. Resistance will be felt when the pin reaches the bottom of the channel.

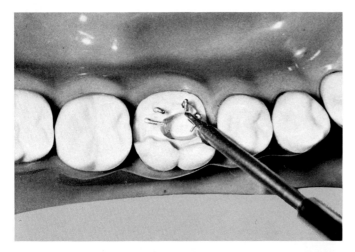

Fig. 14-19 Pins can be bent to bring them within the contour of the core. The force applied to the pin is transmitted through its tip to the tooth structure, and bending the pin can be hazardous.[5] There is less potential for damage to the tooth if pins are merely shortened.

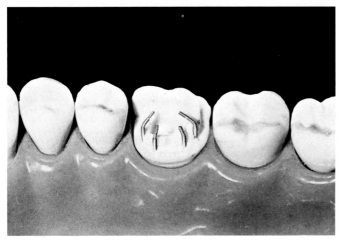

Fig. 14-20 With the pins in place, the tooth is ready to receive the amalgam pin core.

Fig. 14-21 A matrix band is placed around the tooth to contain the amalgam while it is condensed. The type used will depend on the amount of remaining tooth structure to retain the band.

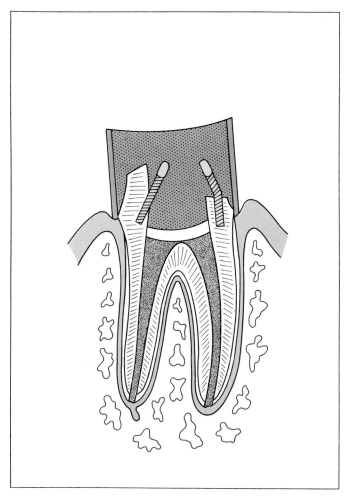

Fig. 14-22 The nearly intact facial surface and supragingival location of most of the finish line permits the use of a Tofflemire matrix here. Both proximal areas have been securely wedged to prevent a gingival overhang. This may not be possible on teeth in which the gingival floor of the proximal box extends subgingivally. Although the proximal contact areas have been burnished in this example, it is not necessary to obtain tight contacts if the crown preparation is to be done soon.

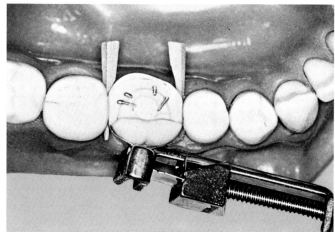

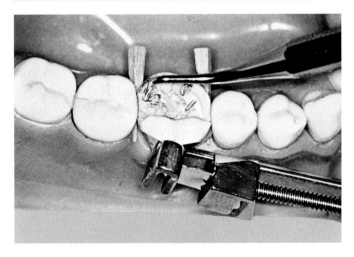

Fig. 14-23   Begin the placement of the amalgam by carefully condensing the material around each pin. The core can be retained by the pins only if it totally surrounds each of them. Avoid hitting the pins too forcefully. It is possible to loosen them.

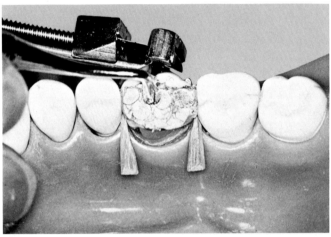

Fig.   14-24   Continue   adding amalgam until the matrix is filled and   the   pins   are   completely covered. Go over the entire occlusal surface with a large amalgam condenser.

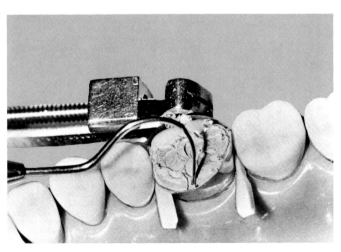

Fig. 14-25   Clear amalgam away from the matrix band by running the tip of an explorer around the inside edge of the matrix band. Occlusal   embrasures   along   the marginal ridges are produced in this way, and the occlusal table can be narrowed.

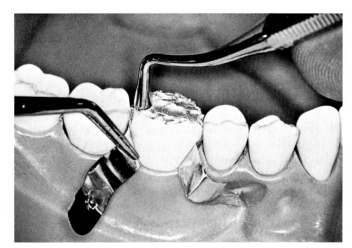

Fig. 14-26 Place the head of a large amalgam condenser on the marginal ridge area to support it while the matrix band is pulled up through the contact area.

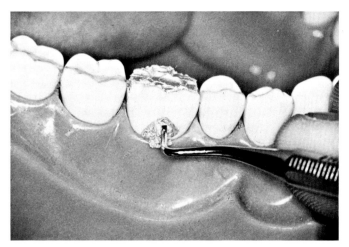

Fig. 14-27 If there are any separate axial areas to be filled in, that should be accomplished now. If the Class V is shallow enough that most of it would be removed when the facial axial reduction is accomplished for the crown preparation, it should be based with polycarboxylate cement at this time. Amalgam is placed only in a preparation deep enough to retain it after the axial reduction has removed some of the surrounding, supporting tooth structure.

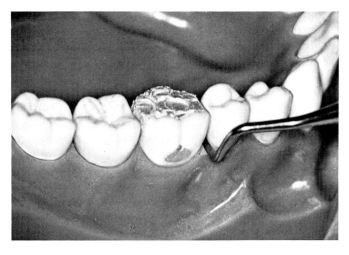

Fig. 14-28 Carefully eliminate any gingival flash that may have extruded past the wedges. A double-ended gold knife works best for this task. Removal of gingival excess makes the crown preparation easier, and it prevents gingival irritation if the amalgam core is to serve for any period of time as a temporary restoration of the tooth.

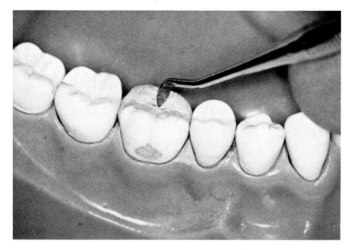

Fig. 14-29 If the crown preparation is to be started soon, the occlusal surface is carved as it would be for the occlusal reduction. If the amalgam will act as a temporary restoration, then it will be left in *light* occlusal contact to prevent supereruption or drifting.

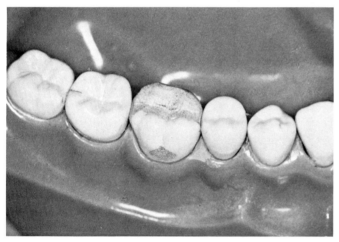

Fig. 14-30 The condensed and carved amalgam pin core is ready to be prepared for the final restoration. The amalgam can serve as an excellent temporary restoration until the crown is started.

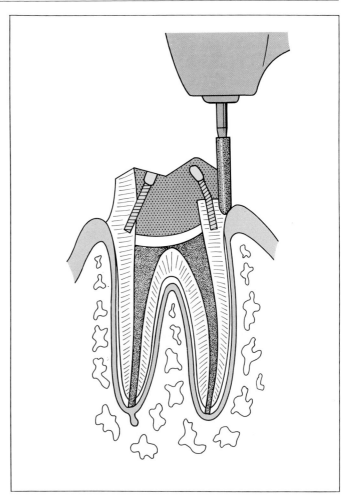

Fig. 14-31 A crown preparation is made on the tooth with the amalgam pin core, treating the amalgam as though it were tooth structure. If the preparation is started at the same appointment in which the amalgam core was placed, use only diamonds on the preparation.

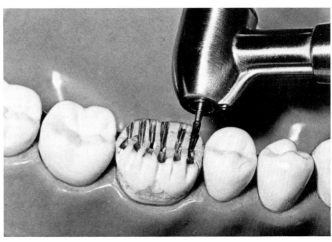

Fig. 14-32 Use depth orientation grooves on the occlusal surface to assure that adequate clearance is obtained.

329

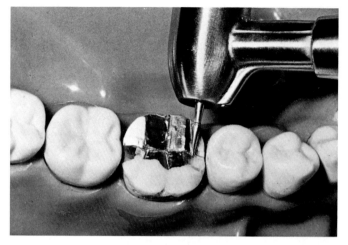

Fig. 14-33 Occlusal reduction is completed by removing the tooth structure between the depth orientation grooves. The geometric inclined plane pattern of the intact occlusal surface is reproduced in the occlusal surface of the crown preparation.

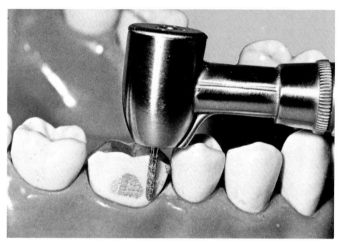

Fig. 14-34 Begin the axial reduction on the facial surface with a chamfer diamond,* carrying the diamond into the facial embrasures as far as possible. If the Class V amalgam were so shallow that it became dislodged, it would be replaced with polycarboxylate to eliminate the undercut.

* No. 877 010 diamond, Brasseler USA Inc., Savannah, GA.

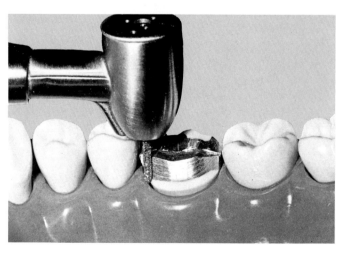

Fig. 14-35 Lingual axial reduction is accomplished with the same instrument. A chamfer finish line is formed as the axial reduction is done.

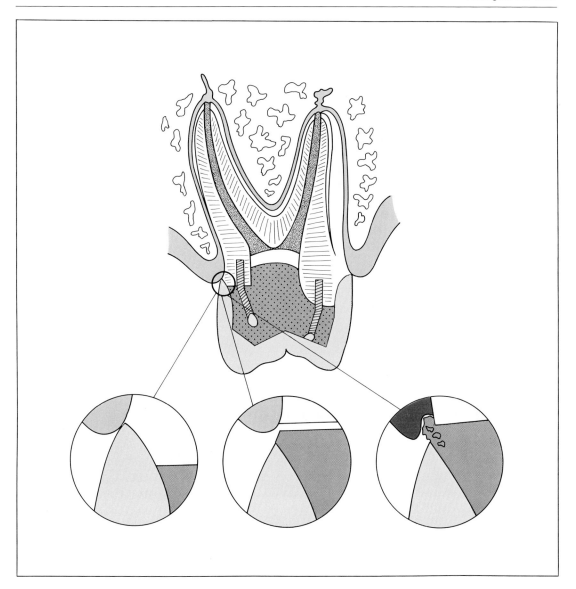

Fig. 14-36 As the preparation is completed, it is important to insure that the preparation finish line for the final restoration be on solid tooth structure, apical to the margin of the amalgam core (left). If it is not possible to verify that the crown margin will cover the margin of the amalgam core, a marginal defect could result. If the finish line is positioned so far apically that the dentist can't determine whether it is on tooth structure or not, it is highly unlikely that the matrix band was very well adapted. As a result, there could be voids in the amalgam at or near the margin (center), or the amalgam could have extruded over the margin (right). If necessary, electrosurgery or periodontal surgery is done to provide access.

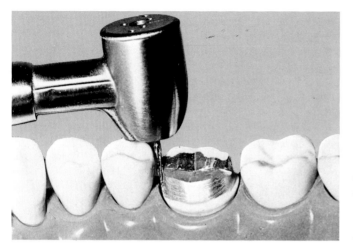

Fig. 14-37 Since there is amalgam in both interproximal areas, a long/thin/tapered bur (No. 169L) is used to produce the initial axial reduction on these surfaces.

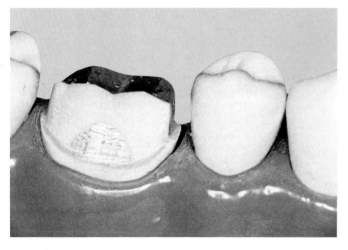

Fig. 14-38 A narrow shoulder, or ledge, is produced simultaneously with the reduction of the proximal surface.

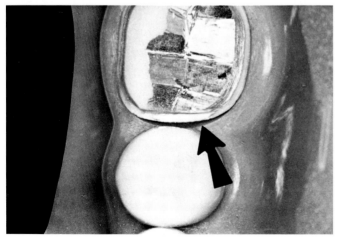

Fig. 14-39 Viewed from the occlusal, the shoulder quickly affords a check on the position of the finish line. Because amalgam is visible on the shoulder (arrow), the finish line obviously still traverses the amalgam core.

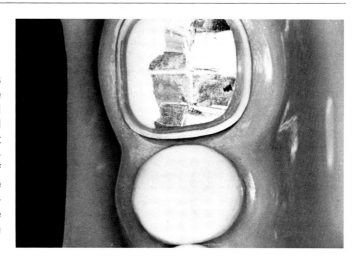

Fig. 14-40 The finish line is lowered farther apically. The tooth constricts mesially and distally as the cemento-enamel junction is approached, making it necessary to do more axial reduction to maintain the width of the shoulder. A check of the shoulder now reveals no amalgam, indicating that the finish line has been moved far enough gingivally.

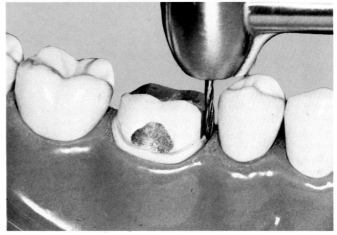

Fig. 14-41 A bevel is added to the proximal shoulder with a chamfer bur.* If the shoulder is wide, the resulting finish line will be a shoulder with a bevel. If it was more of a narrow ledge, it will become a chamfer. Either is a satisfactory finish line for a cast restoration.

* No. 282-010 bur, Brasseler USA Inc., Savannah, GA.

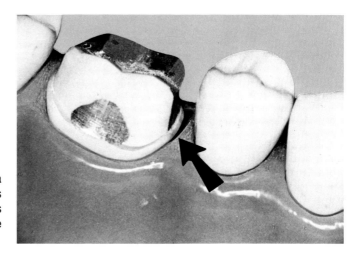

Fig. 14-42 A shoulder with a bevel was produced in this situation (arrow). It blends smoothly into a chamfer on the facial and the lingual.

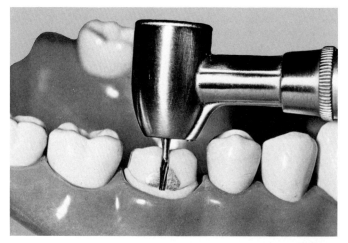

Fig. 14-43 Place a seating groove on the axial surface of the functional cusp with a No. 170 bur. It will end 0.5-1.0 mm. short of the finish line. Its gingival floor should be in tooth structure if at all possible.

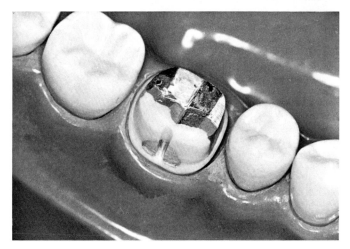

Fig. 14-44 The finished preparation for a full veneer crown preparation has been done on a tooth built-up with an amalgam pin core. Failure to utilize a core would jeopardize the prognosis of the final restoration.

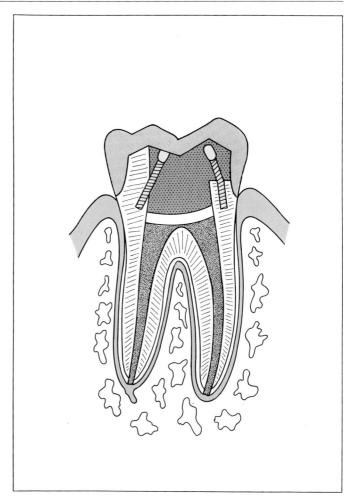

Fig. 14-45 The final restoration will be fabricated over the amalgam core in a routine manner.

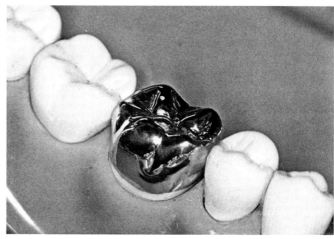

Fig. 14-46 The final restoration for this tooth is a full veneer crown. A porcelain fused to metal restoration can be employed where esthetic requirements are high.

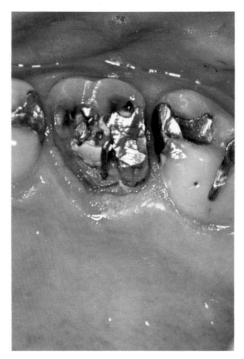

Fig. 14-47 After endodontic treatment, this maxillary molar was built up with an amalgam core which used the silver points obturating the canals as retentive pins. This was compounded by the patient's losing the temporary crown and discontinuing treatment.

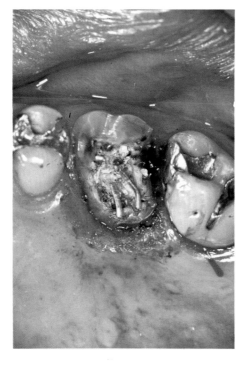

Fig. 14-48 Following retreatment of the root canals, a pin-retained amalgam core was fabricated. Electrosurgery was necessary to uncover the original finish lines in tooth structure. Self-threading pins were used to provide retention for the core.

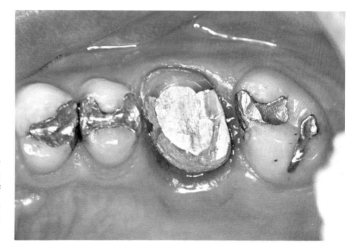

Fig. 14-49 The completed amalgam core and crown preparation are shown before cementation of the final restoration. By using an amalgam core, the restoration has become a routine one.

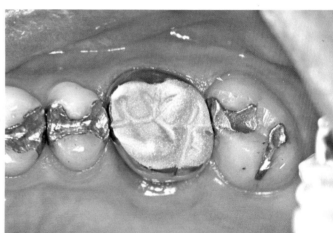

Fig. 14-50 The full crown is seen in the mouth one week after cementation.

References

1. Eissmann, H. F. and Radke, R. A.: Post endodontic restoration. In Cohen, S. and Burns, R. C.: *Pathways of the Pulp.* St. Louis: C. V. Mosby Co., 1976, pp. 537–575.

2. Markley, M. R.: Restorations of silver amalgam. *JADA,* 43:133–146, Aug. 1951.

3. Markley, M. R.: Pin reinforcement and retention of amalgam foundations and restorations. *JADA,* 56:675–679, May 1958.

4. Wing, G.: Pin retention amalgam restorations. *Aust Dent J,* 10:6–10. Feb. 1965.

5. Going, R. E.: Pin retained amalgam. *JADA,* 73:619–624, Sep. 1966.

6. Welk, D. A. and Dilts, W. E.: Influence of pins on the compressive and transverse strength of denal amalgam and retention of pins in amalgam. *JADA,* 78:101–104, Jan. 1969.

7. Collard, E. W., Caputo, A. A. and Standlee, J. P.: Rationale for pin-retained amalgam restorations. *Dent Clin N Amer,* 14:43–51, Jan. 1970.

8. Moffa, J. P., Razzano, M. R. and Doyle, M. G.: Pins – a comparison of their retentive properties. *JADA,* 78:529–535, Mar. 1969.

9. Dilts, W. E., Welk, D. A. and Stovall, J.: Retentive properties of pin materials in pin-retained silver amalgam restorations. *JADA,* 77:1085–1089, Nov. 1968.

10. Caputo, A. A. and Standlee, J. P.: Pins and posts – why, when, and how. *Dent Clin N Amer,* 20:299–311, Apr. 1976.

11. Dilts, W. E., Welk, D. A., Laswell, H. R. and George, L.: Crazing of tooth structure associated with placement of pins for amalgam restorations. *JADA,* 81:387–390, Aug. 1970.

12. Standlee, J. P., Collard, E. W. and Caputo, A. A.: Dentinal defects caused by some twist drills and retentive pins. *J Prosthet Dent,* 24:185–192, Aug. 1970.

13. Johnson, J. K., Schwartz, N. L. and Blackwell, R. T.: Evaluation and restoration of endodontically treated posterior teeth. *JADA,* 93:597–605, Sep. 1976.

14. Chan, K. C., Fuller, J. L. and Khowassah, M. A.: The adaptation of new amalgam and composite resins to pins. *J Prosthet Dent,* 38:392–395, Oct. 1977.

15. Fujimoto, J., Norman, R. D., Dykema, R. W. and Phillips, R. W.: A comparison of pin-retained amalgam and composite resin cores. *J Prosthet Dent,* 39:512–519, May 1978.

16. Roberts, E. W.: Crown reconstruction with pin reinforced amalgam. *Texas Dent J,* 81:10–14, Jun. 1963.

17. Courtade, G. L.: Pin pointers. III. Self-threading pins. *J Prosthet Dent,* 20:335–338, Oct. 1968.

18. Schwartz, N. L.: Restoration of the endodontically treated tooth. 46th Annual Meeting, American Prosthodontic Society, Washington D.C., Nov. 8, 1974.

19. Lerner, T. R., Symons, B. and Schlagel, E.: Restoring and rebuilding the endodontically treated teeth. *NY Dent J,* 32:107–111, Mar. 1966.

20. Watson, R. J.: Amalgam foundations for anterior teeth. *Dent Dig,* 73:206–207, May 1967.

21. Outhwaite, W. C., Garman, T. A. and Pashley, D. H.: Pin vs. slot retention in extensive amalgam restorations. *J Prosthet Dent,* 41:396–400, Apr. 1979.

22. Nayyar, A., Walton, R. E. and Leonard, L. A.: An amalgam coronal-radicular dowel and core technique for endodontically treated posterior teeth. *J Prosthet Dent,* 43:511–515, May 1980.

23. Hormati, A. A. and Denehy, G. E.: Retention of cast crowns cemented to amalgam and composite resin cores. *J Prosthet Dent,* 45:525–528, May 1981.

24. Larson, T. D. and Jensen, J. R.: Microleakage of composite resin and amalgam core material under complete cast crowns. *J Prosthet Dent,* 44:40–44, Jul. 1980.

25. Hormati, A. A. and Denehy, G. E.: Microleakage of pin-retained amalgam and composite resin bases. *J Prosthet Dent,* 44:526–530, Nov. 1980.

26. Lovdahl, P. E. and Nicholls, J. I.: Pin-retained amalgam cores vs. cast gold dowel-cores. *J Prosthet Dent,* 38:507–514, Nov. 1977.

27. Markley, M. R.: Pin retained and reinforced restorations and foundations. *Dent Clin N Amer,* 11:229–244, Mar. 1967.

28. Evans, J. R. and Wetz, J. H.: The pin-amalgam restoration. Part I. A review. *J Prosthet Dent,* 37:37–41, Jan. 1977.

Chapter 15

Composite Resin Pin Core

Composite resin cores have been described for use with different types of dowels. They can also be used with pins in place of amalgam cores for the restoration of molars with some remaining coronal tooth structure. In addition to being easy to manipulate and strong,[1] composite resin has the great advantage of allowing core insertion and crown preparation in one appointment.[1-3] Other types of resin have been used for this purpose,[4] but composites are most popular because of their strength. The resin adapts well to retentive pins,[5] and composite resin cores possess as much tensile strength as amalgam cores.[6] Not one of the resin cores studied by Fujimoto and associates failed by the core separating from the pins. Pin-retained composite cores have been found by some investigators to be equal,[7] or superior,[8] to cast dowel-cores in resistance to displacement.

On the negative side, composite resin cores exhibit greater microleakage than do amalgam cores.[9] When this is coupled with the observation that crowns cemented to cores, amalgam or resin, leak more than crowns cemented to tooth structure,[10] there is a strong potential for leakage into the canal. This finding is given credence by the clinical recommendation that the crown margin be on tooth structure, well removed from the margin of the core.[11-13] Composite resin cores show less tensile bond strength for cast crowns than do amalgam cores at the time of cementation. The retentive capability of the composite resin cores increases with time, however.[14] There is also some indication that the surface of composite resin is altered by cements containing eugenol.[15]

What is the clinical significance of these phenomena? Since the material has not been in use for very long, it is difficult to assess at this point. Very possibly there is no clinical significance at all.

If composite resin cores are to be used with these questions still unanswered, certain precautions would be prudent. Crown margins should extend well past core margins. The composite resin core should not extend down into the pulp chamber or root canal. Composite resin cores should be employed only in the build-up of teeth to receive single crowns. Bridge abutments should be built-up in some other way. Temporary crowns on teeth with composite resin cores should be cemented with some cement other than zinc oxide-eugenol. Obviously, the teeth should be covered with well fitting temporary crowns. The core itself should not be used as a temporary restoration.

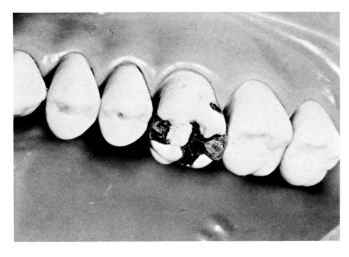

Fig. 15-1 An endodontically treated maxillary molar with a large existing amalgam and further damage inflicted by caries and decalcification would be a good indication for a pin-retained composite resin core if it still had sound coronal tooth structure.

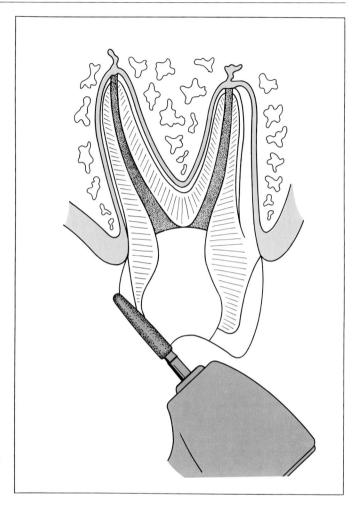

Fig. 15-2 Old bases, caries, and undermined tooth structure are removed for the fabrication of a composite resin pin core.

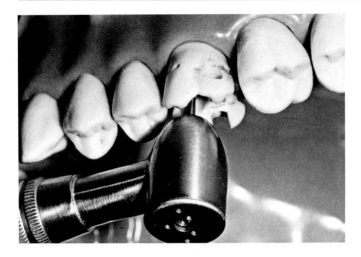

Fig. 15-3 Remove all the bases down to the covering over the pulp chamber. Because of the possibility of microleakage, do *not* extend the preparation into the pulp chamber itself.

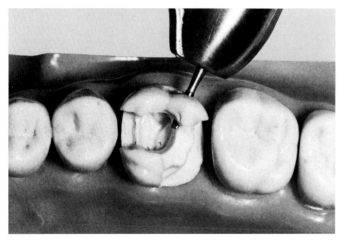

Fig. 15-4 Follow any communicating tracts between the old preparation and newly excavated caries. If "islands" of isolated and poorly supported tooth structure, such as this distobuccal cusp, are created, they should be eliminated.

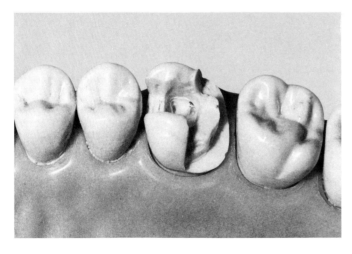

Fig. 15-5 Removal of all caries and compromised tooth structure has eliminated the two distal cusps. The presence of the two mesial cusps, with underlying dentin and a bulk of tooth structure around the core of the tooth, would permit the use of a pin-retained composite resin core.

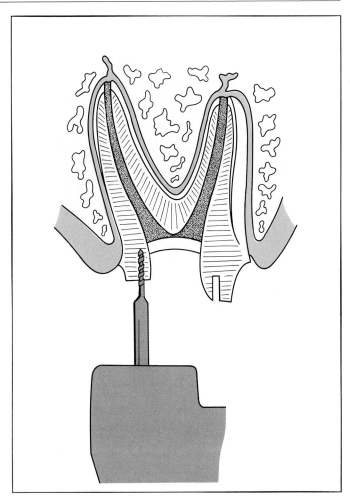

Fig. 15-6 Place the pin holes in areas where there is some bulk. Favor the dentino-enamel junction, moving closer to the pulp with the pin holes. This should lessen dentinal crazing and eliminate any chance of lateral perforation.

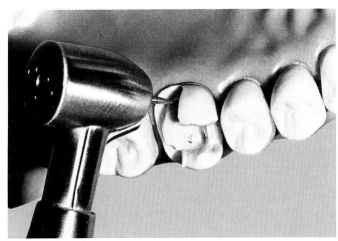

Fig. 15-7 All pin holes are started with a No. ½ round bur to permit exact placement of the channel. If the initial penetration is attempted with a twist drill, it may skip or slide.

343

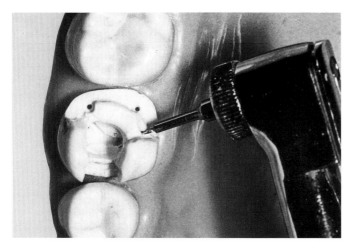

Fig. 15-8 The actual pin holes are made with a twist drill. A 0.5 mm. drill is used if the Minim pin is to provide the retention. Prepare the hole with a minimum number of insertions and withdrawals to avoid overenlarging it. Mark the vial in which the drill is stored to record the number of holes placed with it. Discard the drill after 20 holes.[16]

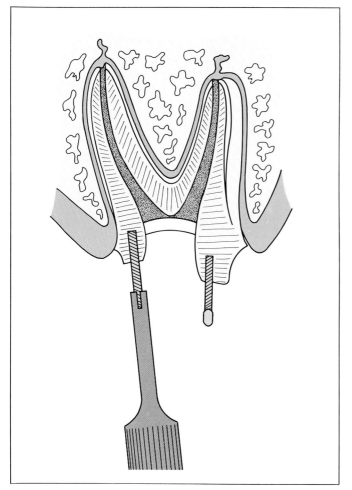

Fig. 15-9 Place the pins in their holes with a light touch. Avoid overseating them since this generates stress and causes microfracture of the dentin.

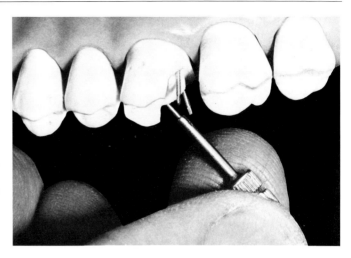

Fig. 15-10 A hand wrench is employed where access will permit it. This provides a sensory precaution against overtorquing the pin. To prevent a build-up of stress, stop threading the pin as soon as any slight resistance is felt.

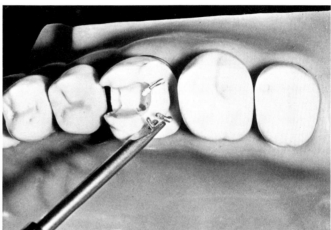

Fig. 15-11 Although a pin can be bent to position it within the eventual contours of the composite resin core, this should be done sparingly. It can fracture the tooth if it is too near the periphery or surrounded by thin, weak tooth structure. The pin can also be stripped out of its hole. The pin can be shortened to achieve the same result in many situations.

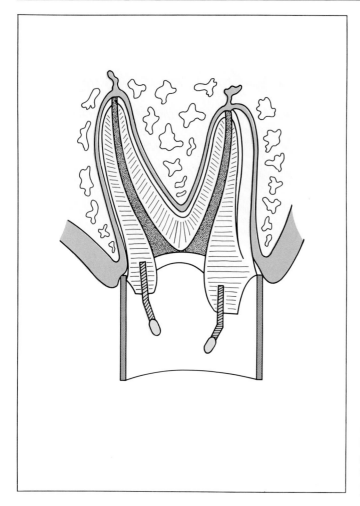

Fig. 15-12 When the pins have been placed, a matrix of some sort is positioned around the tooth to hold the resin when it is put in the preparation.

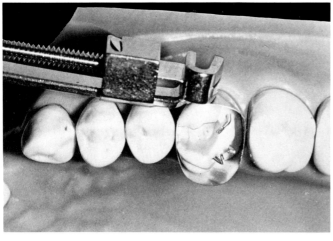

Fig. 15-13 A Tofflemire matrix can be used to contain the composite resin during insertion. Lubricated polycarbonate crowns have also been used as matrices.[17]

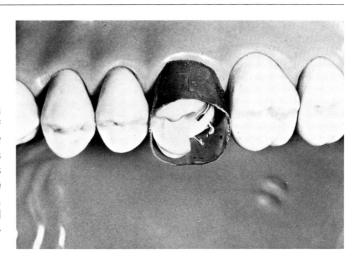

Fig. 15-14 A copper band is ideally suited for the placement of composite resin cores. To allow better adaptation to the tooth, it is festooned to follow the contours of the gingiva. No effort is made to burnish the proximal contacts, since the crown preparation will be done at the same appointment.

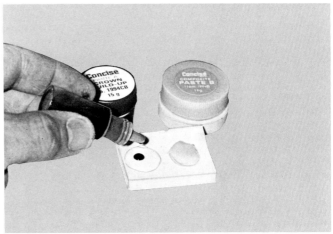

Fig. 15-15 Trim off a Centrix syringe tip to produce a large opening to accommodate the bulk of resin needed to make a core. Mix a large quantity of an opaque composite material.*
To increase color contrast and visibility, add a small drop of green food coloring to the mix.

* Concise Crown Build-Up Material, 3-M Dental Products, St. Paul, MN.

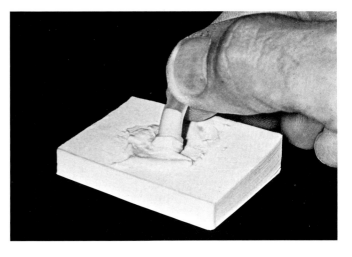

Fig. 15-16 Load the composite resin into the syringe tip by running the back end of the plastic tip across the mixing pad. Place the conical rubber plunger in the tip behind the resin, and insert the tip into the metal syringe.

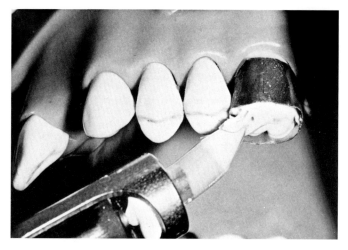

Fig. 15-17 The resin is injected forcefully from a Centrix C-R syringe.* Make sure that it completely surrounds every retention pin and fills all recessed areas of the preparation.

* Centrix C-R Syringe, Centrix Inc., Hartford, CT.

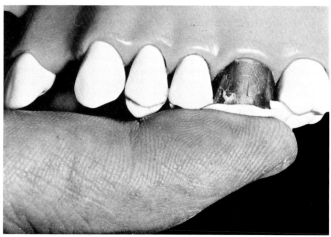

Fig. 15-18 When the matrix is overflowing, clamp a fingertip over the end of the matrix to compress the resin around the pins and into every possible undercut in the preparation.

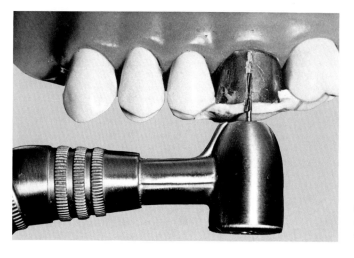

Fig. 15-19 Use a bur in the high speed handpiece to section the copper band and make it easier to remove.

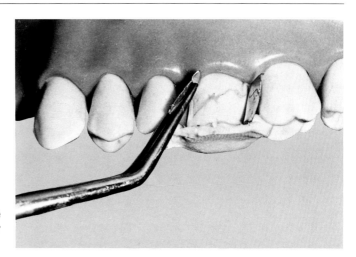

Fig. 15-20 Peel the band off the tooth with cotton pliers or mosquito forceps.

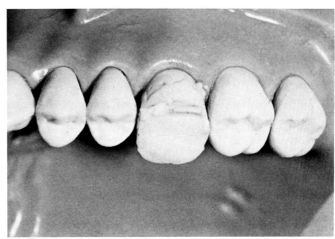

Fig. 15-21 The composite resin core is the size and general shape of the tooth to be restored. The pin-retained blank can easily be shaped to the contours of a crown preparation.

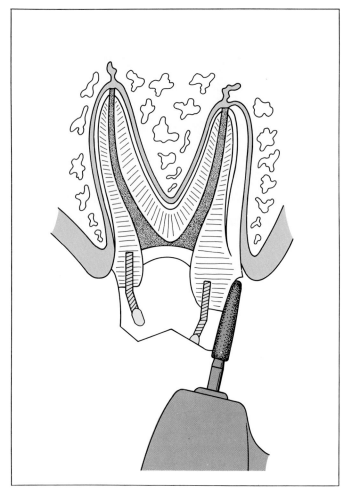

Fig. 15-22 The crown preparation is begun as soon as the matrix is removed. Diamonds are used because they are more effective in cutting the composite resin.

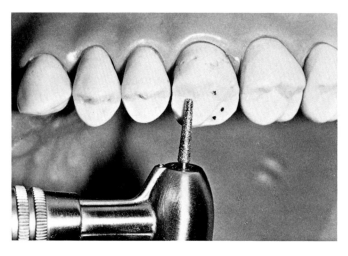

Fig. 15-23 Occlusal reduction is accomplished first, using a round-end or flat-end tapered diamond. A minimum of 1.5 mm. clearance should be obtained over the entire occlusal surface.

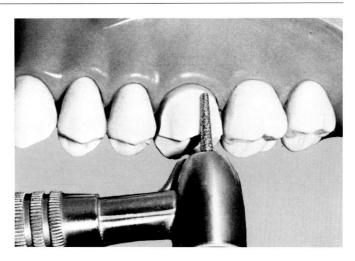

Fig. 15-24 A flat-end tapered diamond is used for the facial axial reduction of the porcelain fused to metal restoration. A shoulder finish line is formed simultaneously. It will be at least 1.0 mm. wide, with the facial reduction being somewhat deeper near the occlusal surface.

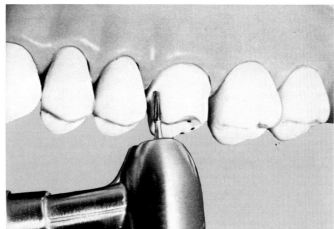

Fig. 15-25 Finish the facial reduction and shoulder with a No. 170 bur. It may be necessary to use a No. 10-4-8 hoe on the shoulder to smooth it.

Fig. 15-26 Proximal axial reduction is started with a short, thin tapered diamond* small enough to maneuver in a restricted area. Lingual axial reduction is done with a chamfer diamond** which is extended through the interproximal areas to connect with the facial shoulder.

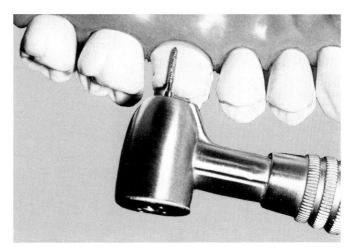

* No. 852-012 diamond, Brasseler, USA Inc., Savannah, GA.
** No. 887-010 diamond, Brasseler, USA Inc., Savannah, GA.

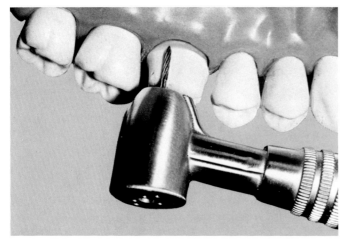

Fig. 15-27 Smooth the axial reduction and chamfer finish line with a chamfer bur.* This carbide finishing bur will produce a definite, well instrumented finish line.

* No. 282-010 bur, Brasseler USA Inc., Savannah, GA.

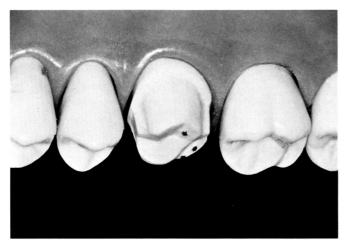

Fig. 15-28 The completed porcelain fused to metal crown preparation utilizes the pin-retained composite resin core to make up deficiencies in both contour and retention that occurred when the distal cusps were lost.

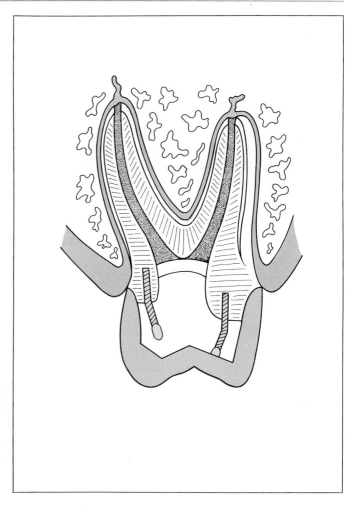

Fig. 15-29 The fabrication of a porcelain fused to metal crown over the composite resin pin core progresses in a normal manner. The impression for the final restoration is made during the same appointment at which the resin core was fabricated.

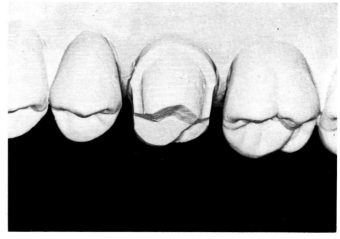

Fig. 15-30 The cast poured from the final impression is ready for fabrication of the crown. The preparation made from a core will be remarkable only because it will have fewer compromises and flaws than a preparation done only in natural tooth structure.

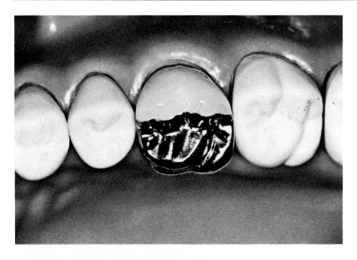

Fig. 15-31 The completed porcelain fused to metal crown is cemented over a maxillary molar with a pin-retained composite resin core.

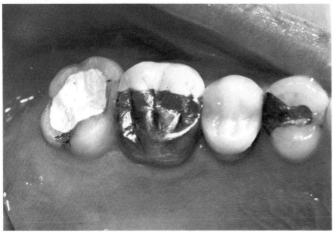

Fig. 15-32 There were significant quantities of tooth structure under the two mesial cusps of this maxillary molar, although the tooth was rather short.

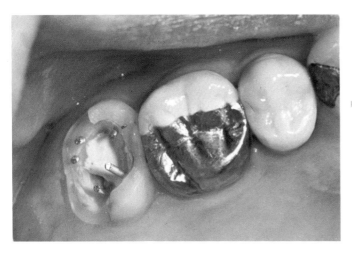

Fig. 15-33 After the polycarboxylate temporary restoration was removed, the extent of the core could be assessed. Four pins were placed, since they could not be the optimum 2.0 mm. in length. Notice that polycarboxylate cement still covers the pulp chamber.

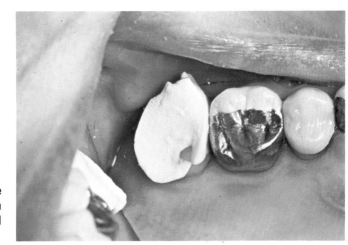

Fig. 15-34 The composite core is seen after insertion. The crown preparation has not been started yet.

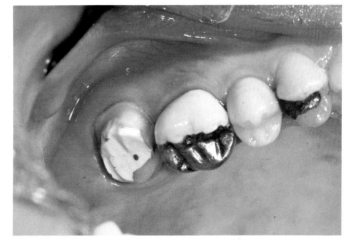

Fig. 15-35 The completed porcelain fused to metal crown preparation is seen on the maxillary second molar. Although coloring was not added to the core, the opaque white composite resin makes differentiation of tooth structure and core a relatively simple task.

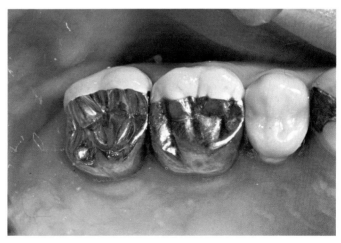

Fig. 15-36 The porcelain fused to metal crown is cemented over the pin-retained composite resin core.

References

1. Spalten, R. G.: Composite resins to restore multilated teeth. *J Prosthet Dent,* 25:323–326, Mar. 1971.

2. Schmidt, J. R., Ehrenkranz, H., Mohamed, S. E. and Franklin, M. E.: A single visit post and core procedure. *NY St Dent J,* 39:604–610, Dec. 1973.

3. Landwerlen, J. R. and Berry, H. H.: Composite resin post and core. *J Prosthet Dent,* 28:500–503, Nov. 1972.

4. Shulman, L. S.: Plastic pin cores. *Dent Dig,* 76:429–430, Oct. 1970.

5. Chan, K. C., Fuller, J. L. and Khowassah, M. A.: The adaptation of new amalgam and composite resins to pins. *J Prosthet Dent,* 38:392–395, Oct. 1977.

6. Fujimoto, J., Norman, R. D., Dykema, R. W. and Phillips, R. W.: A comparison of pin-retained amalgam and composite resin cores. *J Prosthet Dent,* 39:512–519, May 1978.

7. Newburg, R. E. and Pameijer, C. H.: Retentive properties of post and core systems. *J Prosthet Dent,* 36:636–643, Dec. 1976.

8. Perez-Moll, J. F., Howe, D. F. and Svare, C. W.: Cast gold post and core and pin-retained composite resin bases: A comparative study in strength. *J Prosthet Dent,* 40:642–644, Dec. 1978.

9. Hormati, A. A. and Denehy, G. E.: Microleakage of pin-retained amalgam and composite resin bases. *J Prosthet Dent,* 44:526–530, Nov. 1980.

10. Larson, T. D. and Jensen, J. R.: Microleakage of composite resin and amalgam core material under complete cast crowns. *J Prosthet Dent,* 44:40–44, July 1980.

11. Eissmann, H. F. and Radke, R. A.: Post endodontic restoration. In Cohen, S. and Burns, R. C.: *Pathways of the Pulp.* St. Louis: C.V. Mosby Co., 1976, pp. 537–575.

12. Johnson, J. K., Schwartz, N. L. and Blackwell, R. T.: Evaluation and restoration of endodontically treated posterior teeth. *JADA,* 93:597–605, Sep. 1976.

13. Fagin, M. D.: Restoration of endodontically treated teeth. *Int J Periodont Rest Dent,* 1(3):9–29, 1981.

14. Hormati, A. A. and Denehy, G. E.: Retention of cast crowns cemented to amalgam and composite resin cores. *J Prosthet Dent,* 45:525–528, May 1981.

15. Millstein, P. L. and Nathanson, D.: Effects of eugenol and eugenol containing cements on cured composite resin. *J Dent Res,* Abstract No. 633, 1980.

16. Standlee, J. P., Collard, E. W. and Caputo, A. A.: Dentinal defects caused by some twist drills and retentive pins. *J Prosthet Dent,* 24:185–192, Aug. 1970.

17. Light, E. I., Chertoff, A. and Rakow, B.: Simultaneous fabrication of a core and temporary crown. *Dent Surv,* 50:36–39, Jul. 1974.

Chapter 16

Temporary Restorations for Endodontically Treated Teeth

A temporary restoration commonly plays an important role in the successful restoration of a tooth. It is true that the normally essential role of pulpal protection is not of concern in dealing with an endodontically treated tooth. Nevertheless, the temporary restoration may be even more important to the patient receiving a dowel-core and a crown. The loss of all tooth structure visible to the patient is traumatic in itself, especially if it has occurred suddenly.

In addition to its important esthetic role, the temporary restoration also serves other functions. It protects the tooth from further damage, prevents the migration of adjacent contacting teeth, and provides occlusal function.[1]

The biggest problem in fabricating a temporary restoration is the same one encountered in restoring the endodontically treated tooth in the first place. Some substitute must be found for the lost tooth structure, so a form of dowel-crown is usually employed.

A number of different crown formers and dowels are used in various combinations. Polycarbonate crowns have been relined with acrylic,[2-5] as have celluloid crown forms.[6] Overimpressions[3, 4, 7] and plastic shells[8, 9] have also been used to form the outer contours of the crown. An effort is usually made to get some acrylic into the canal. While there may be nothing but acrylic in the canal,[6, 9] it is often reinforced with wire.[3, 7, 8] Other types of retentive devices have included plastic dowels relined with acrylic resin,[5] a silicone dowel reinforced with a paper clip,[1] metal dowels with no acrylic lining,[2, 3] and a wooden match stick.[10] Some prefabricated dowel systems have steel dowels made specifically for temporary crowns. However, they work best if the matching reamer was used in preparing the canal for the final dowel-core.

The polycarbonate crown is well suited for the routine single crown. If the temporary restoration involves a bridge, or unusual alignment or morphology in a single crown, a custom plastic shell will probably provide the best result in the shortest time.

357

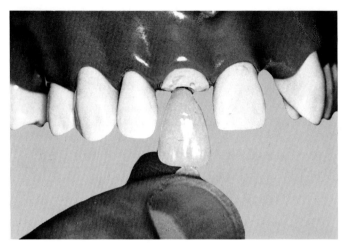

Polycarbonate Crown

Fig. 16-1 The polycarbonate crown is used with a paper clip dowel to provide temporary coverage for the endodontically treated tooth. The coronal portion of the restoration is composed of a polycarbonate crown form, relined with acrylic resin. Initially, a crown is chosen that has dimensions compatible with the space it will occupy.

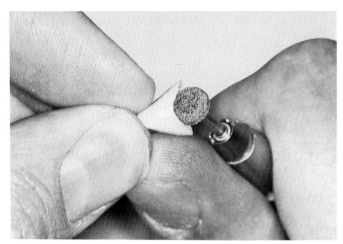

Fig. 16-2 In most cases, the crown will not adapt around the existing root without modification. Excess length is removed from the gingival margin of the crown, while the incisal area is left intact.

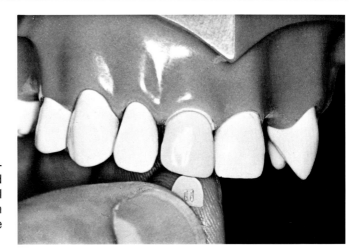

Fig. 16-3 This process is con-
tinued until the crown is adapted
reasonably well to the gingival
finish line, with the incisal edge in
the proper position relative to the
adjacent teeth.

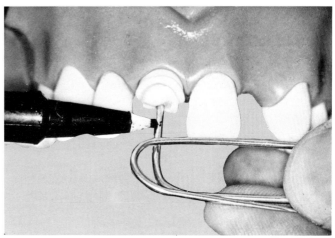

Fig. 16-4 A section of paper clip
made of heavy gauge wire is
placed into the canal to its full
depth. A felt tip pen mark is
placed 2-4 mm. above the remaining coronal tooth structure.
The length of wire extending into
the crown will be dictated by the
length of the crown. The longer
the exposed piece of paper clip,
the better its retention in the
acrylic resin in the crown.

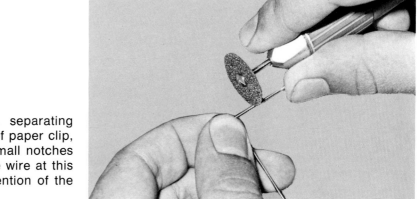

Fig. 16-5 Using a separating
disc, cut the length of paper clip,
as marked. Some small notches
can be placed in the wire at this
time to assist in retention of the
resin.

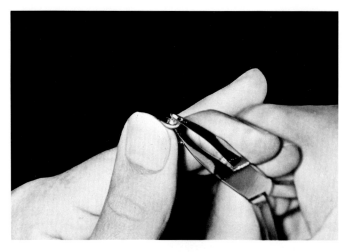

Fig. 16-6 Place a bend near the end of the wire. When embedded in the temporary crown, this bend will prevent the dowel from pulling out and rotating.

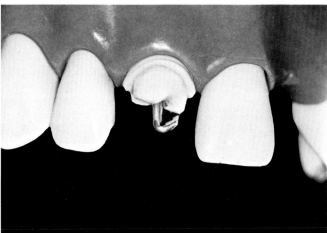

Fig. 16-7 Try the trimmed dowel in the canal and confirm that the polycarbonate crown will have room to seat without binding on the wire.

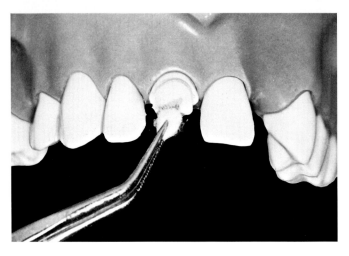

Fig. 16-8 The root face is lightly lubricated with petrolatum to prevent any acrylic resin from sticking to the tooth during polymerization.

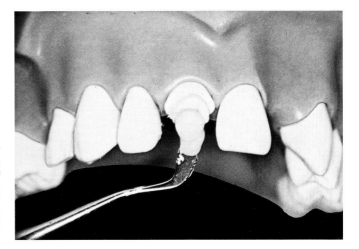

Fig. 16-9 A thin mix of temporary acrylic resin is placed on the root face around the orifice of the canal. Avoid placing any resin deep into the canal space itself, since this can make the crown difficult to remove.

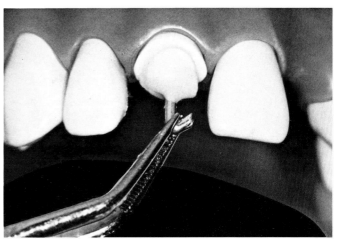

Fig. 16-10 Insert the paper clip dowel into the canal.

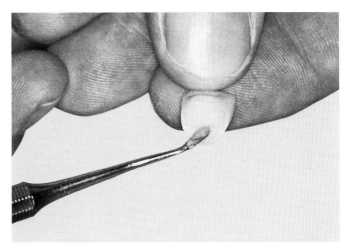

Fig. 16-11 Fill the polycarbonate crown with the same mix of acrylic resin. Eliminate any voids in the material before placing it on the tooth.

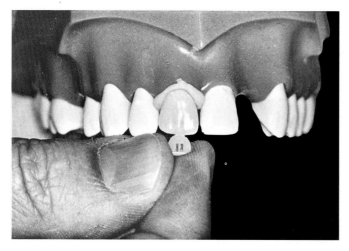

Fig. 16-12 Seat the crown and confirm that it is in the proper position relative to the adjacent teeth. Excess acrylic can be removed with an explorer to make trimming easier. As the material reaches a doughy consistency, the crown should be pumped in and out of the tooth several times to avoid being locked in place during polymerization.

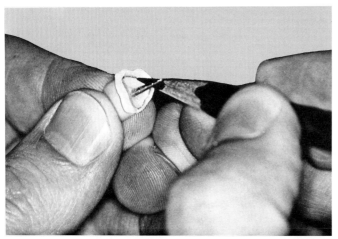

Fig. 16-13 The pin-temporary crown can be placed in hot water to speed polymerization. Prior to trimming and contouring, it is helpful to mark the margin on the inside of the crown with a sharp pencil.

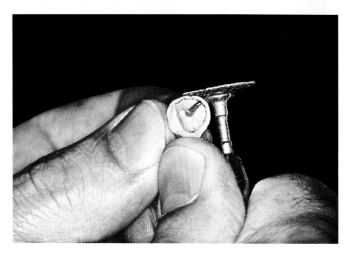

Fig. 16-14 The temporary crown is trimmed with sandpaper discs. The polycarbonate crown will frequently be overcontoured in the gingival one-third. Special attention should be given to properly shaping the restoration and making any needed adjustments in occlusion. Perforating the polycarbonate crown is not a problem because there is an underlying bulk of acrylic.

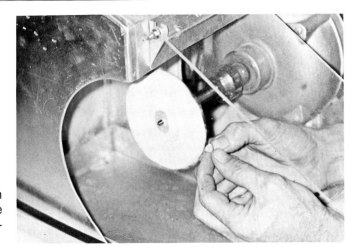

Fig. 16-15 The temporary crown is first polished with fine pumice and then with a high-lustre denture polish.

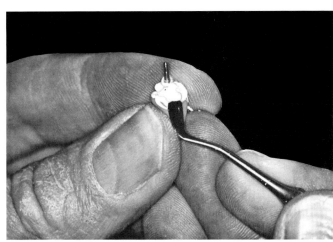

Fig. 16-16 Temporary cement should be placed only in the coronal portion of the restoration. Avoid getting cement in the canal space. A zinc oxide-eugenol cement mixed with an equal part of petrolatum is acceptable.

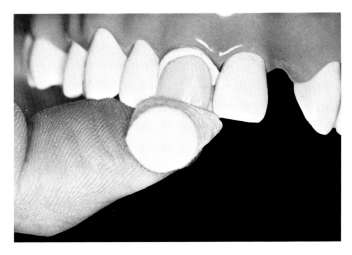

Fig. 16-17 Seat the pin-temporary crown and hold it in place with firm finger pressure until the cement is set.

363

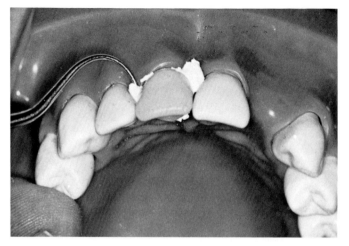

Fig. 16-18 Carefully clean the excess cement from around the margins. Cement left in the sulcus at this point will cause gingival problems that can make impressions at the next appointment difficult or impossible.

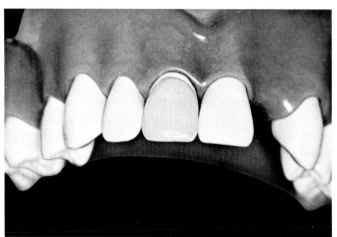

Fig. 16-19 The completed temporary restoration will predictably serve the patient until the permanent dowel-core is delivered. At that time, the wire dowel and acrylic are cut out and the crown can be relined and placed over the dowel-core.

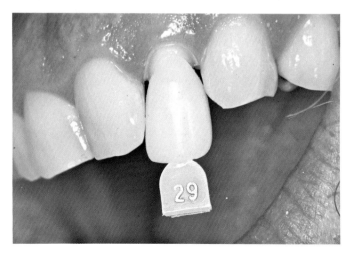

Fig. 16-20 A polycarbonate crown was selected for this maxillary lateral incisor. Some contouring and trimming were needed before relining.

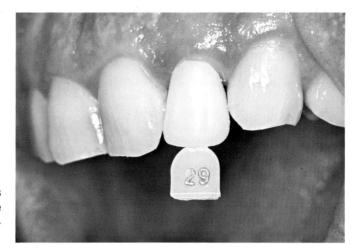

Fig. 16-21 The crown was adapted and trimmed to fit the tooth and blend in with the adjacent teeth.

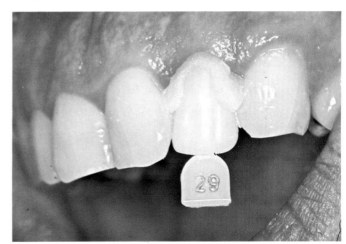

Fig. 16-22 After trimming the paper clip, the acrylic-filled temporary crown was seated.

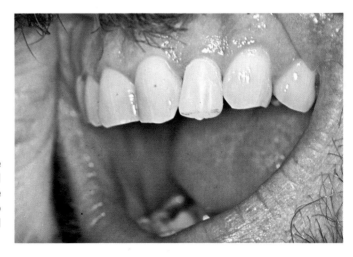

Fig. 16-23 Upon removal of the handling tag, the incisal edge did not quite harmonize with the adjacent teeth. It was slightly too long, especially in its distal aspect.

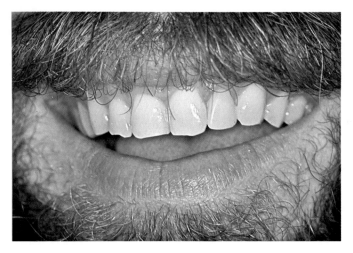

Fig. 16-24   The temporary restoration was cemented, after final contouring and polishing. It met the esthetic and functional demands during the time that the final dowel-core was being fabricated.

Clear Plastic Shell

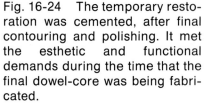

Fig. 16-25   Another method for constructing a pin-temporary crown involves the use of a clear plastic shell. While the shell can be shaped by a vacuum forming machine, it is more easily and economically adapted by using silicone putty.* Begin by placing the putty into an unperforated stock metal impression tray.

* Silly Putty, Binney and Smith, Inc., Easton, PA.

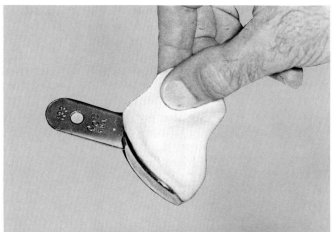

Fig. 16-26   Cut a sheet of coping material* in half and place it in a wire frame, shiny side down. The plastic material is slowly heated over a flame until it sags. If it is translucent, it should become clear as it softens. If the material is the clear variety, it should be heated until it begins to smoke slightly.

* Coping, material, .020 inches, Omnident Corporation, Chicago, IL.

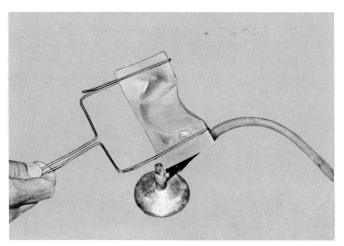

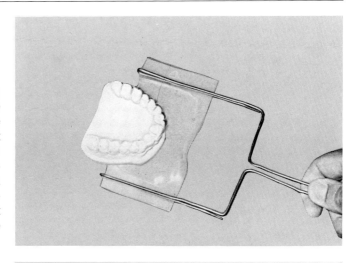

Fig. 16-27 The heated coping material is quickly carried to the diagnostic cast. If the tooth to be restored is badly broken down, it should have been waxed to an acceptable contour and duplicated in plaster or stone. A duplicate cast is necessary because the hot plastic would melt the wax if it were placed on the original cast.

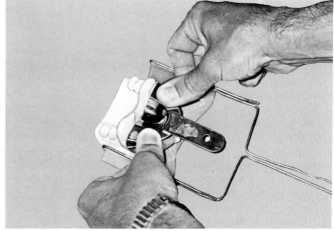

Fig. 16-28 The tray loaded with putty is placed over the plastic and firmly seated on the cast. Compressed air can be blown on the shell to speed cooling.

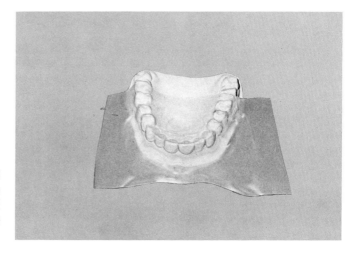

Fig. 16-29 After about 30 seconds, the tray and the silicone putty are removed. A well adapted plastic shell covers the cast.

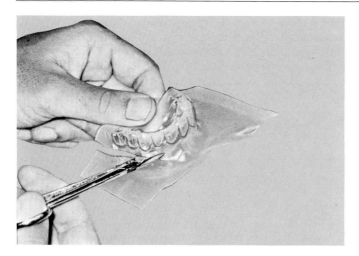

Fig. 16-30 The coping material is removed from the cast and trimmed with scissors.

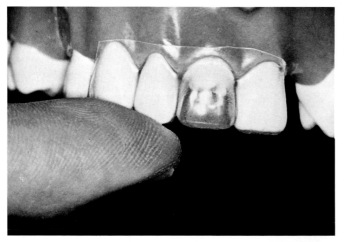

Fig. 16-31 The finished shell should extend at least one tooth in either direction from the tooth being restored. It should also be trimmed to extend no more than 2-3 mm. beyond the gingival sulcus.

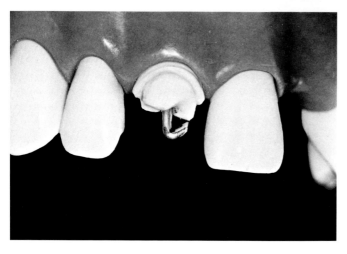

Fig. 16-32 A paper clip is prepared in the same manner described previously. The end is bent to aid retention in the temporary crown.

Fig. 16-33 The shell is filled with temporary acrylic resin. An effort should be made to keep the material in the area of the tooth being restored. If the acrylic runs into adjacent teeth, it can make the shell difficult to seat completely.

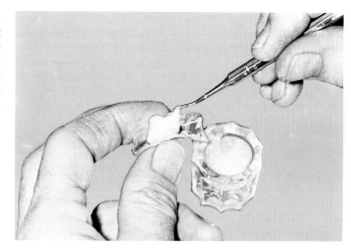

Fig. 16-34 Before seating the shell, examine the acrylic from the outside to make sure there are no obvious voids or bubbles. They can be eliminated much more easily at this time than they can be filled in later. If the mold appears adequately filled, the shell can be seated. Make sure that it is in the proper position by firmly pressing on the incisal edges of the adjacent teeth. Avoid pushing on the tooth being restored because the coping material may overseat and distort the temporary crown.

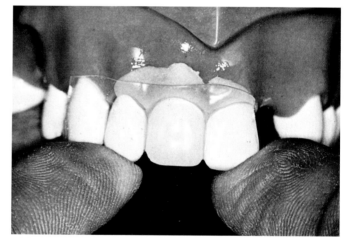

Fig. 16-35 When the material reaches a doughy consistency, remove the shell and separate it from the temporary crown. If it is left in place too long, it can be locked in place in the canal or between adjacent teeth.

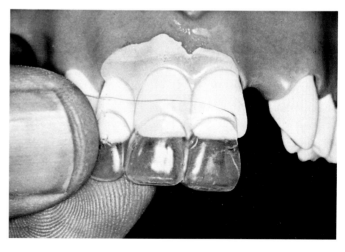

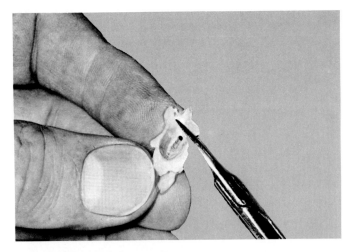

Fig. 16-36 Trim off as much flash as possible with scissors while the acrylic is still doughy. Reseat the crown on the tooth and remove it. Drop the temporary crown in a bowl of hot water to speed polymerization.

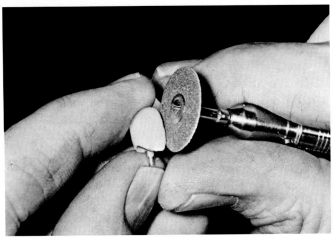

Fig. 16-37 The temporary crown is contoured with a sandpaper disc. Check the occlusion and adjust as necessary. Polish the crown first with pumice and then with high lustre denture polish.

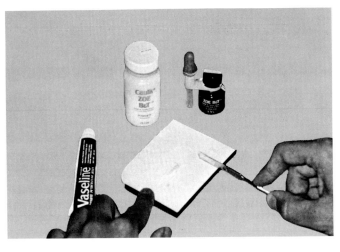

Fig. 16-38 A thin mix of zinc oxide and eugenol with petrolatum is used to cement the pin-temporary crown.

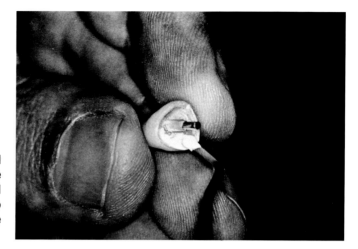

Fig. 16-39 Coat only the coronal areas with cement, avoiding the dowel. If the canal space is filled with cement, it is difficult both to remove the crown and clean the canal.

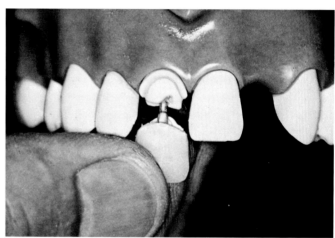

Fig. 16-40 Seat the temporary crown and hold it in place with firm finger pressure until the cement has set.

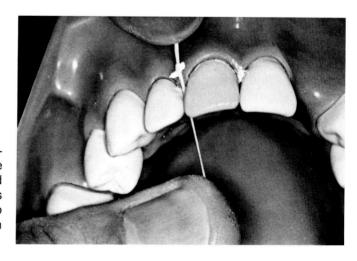

Fig. 16-41 This type of temporary restoration should provide the necessary protection and esthetics while the dowel-core is being fabricated. Be sure to remove all excess cement from the gingival sulcus.

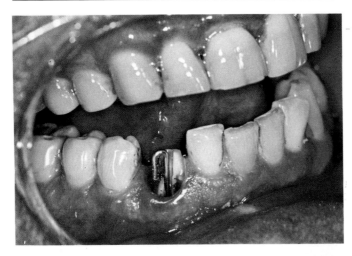

Fig. 16-42   A piece of paper clip wire with a loop in the end was inserted in a mandibular canine.

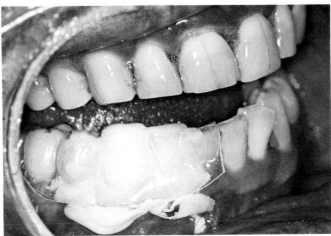

Fig. 16-43   Acrylic was formed with a clear plastic shell.

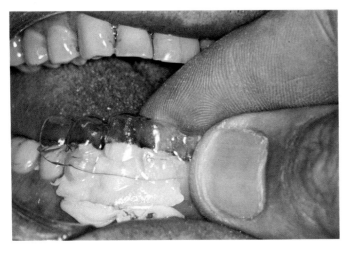

Fig. 16-44   When the acrylic reached a doughy stage, first the shell and then the acrylic were removed from the mouth.

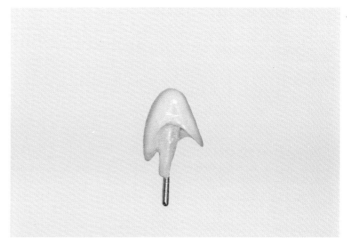

Fig. 16-45 The finished pin-temporary crown shows the reinforcing role played by the wire. It extends the full length of the canal.

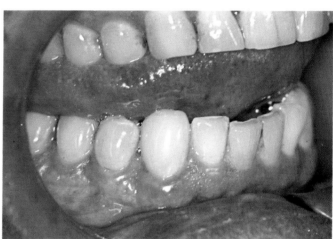

Fig. 16-46 The pin-temporary crown was cemented in place with a diluted zinc oxide-eugenol cement.

References

1. Baraban, D. J.: The restoration of pulpless teeth. *Dent Clin N Amer,* 12:633–653, Nov. 1967.

2. Album, M. M. and Lloyd, R. W.: Technique for restoring endodontically treated teeth with precision posts and porcelain-bonded-to-gold crowns. *JADA,* 93:591–596, Sep. 1976.

3. Hannah, C. McD.: Prefabricated post and core patterns. *J Prosthet Dent,* 30:37–42, Jul. 1973.

4. Holt, J. K.: Anterior post crowns. *Brit Dent J,* 113:299–304, Nov. 1962.

5. Waldman, P. M.: Esthetic temporary crowns for devitalized teeth utilizing a resin post. *Dent Dig,* 74:470–471, Nov. 1968.

6. Baumhammers, A.: Simplified technique for a one-unit cast dowel crown. *Dent Dig,* 68:468–472, Oct. 1962.

7. Dooley, B. S.: Preparation and construction of post-retention crowns for anterior teeth. *Aust Dent J,* 12:544–550, Dec. 1967.

8. Michnick, B. T. and Raskin, R. B.: A multiple post-core technique. *J Prosthet Dent,* 39:622–626, Jun. 1978.

9. Wiland, L.: A dimension controlled and accurate procedure for a gold post restoration of an anterior tooth. *Dent Dig,* 72:394–397, Sep. 1966.

10. Yuodelis, R. and Morrison, K.: Full coverage restoration of pulpless anterior and bicuspid teeth. *J Canad Dent Assoc,* 32:516–521, Sept. 1966.

Authors Index

A

Abdullah, S. I.	20, 24, 96, 143
Abou-Rass, M.	17, 26
Album, M. M.	357
Angmar-Mansson, B.	292
Antonoff, S. J.	20, 24, 33
Arvidson, K.	44
Asawa, G. N.	20, 123
Azarmehr, P.	22, 123

B

Baker, C. R.	20
Bangs, A. S.	95, 96
Baraban, D. J.	15, 16, 75, 79, 164, 228, 357
Barak, M. A.	44
Barker, B. C. W.	15, 20, 33, 45, 53
Barouch, E.	44
Bartlett, S. O.	15, 20, 45
Baum, L.	16, 34, 181, 227
Baumhammers, A.	13, 20, 34, 75, 357
Beheshti, N.	123
Berbert, A.	20, 45
Bergman, M.	205
Berry, H. H.	339
Bjorndal, A. M.	96
Black, G. V.	13
Blair, H. A.	16
Blass, M. S.	20, 205, 211
Borden, B. G.	44
Bower, R. C.	16, 45, 95, 96, 123, 143
Burnell, S. C.	20, 75, 205

C

Caputo, A. A.	15, 17, 19, 24, 25, 26, 27, 28, 29, 33, 63, 163, 164, 181, 240, 241, 253, 258, 260, 267, 275, 291, 292, 313, 314, 322, 344
Chan, K. C.	314, 339
Charbeneau, G. T.	16
Charlton, G.	24, 34, 205
Chertoff, A.	346
Christy, J. M.	20, 24, 205
Clarke, J.	13

Collard, E. W.	25, 28, 33, 63, 181, 253, 258, 260, 267, 313, 314, 322, 344
Colley, I. T.	19, 24, 25, 28, 163
Colman, H. L.	33
Combe, E. C.	258
Courtade, G. L.	314, 322

D

Dale, J. W.	45
Davy, D. T.	44
Dawson, P. E.	15
Day, R. C.	44
DeDomenico, R. J.	45
Demas, N. C.	13, 20
Denehy, G. E.	314, 339
Derand, T.	292
Dewhirst, R. B.	15, 20, 33, 45, 53
Didea, A.	253
Dill, G. C.	45
Dilley, G. L.	44
Dilts, W. E.	313, 314
Dooley, B. S.	15, 20, 24, 34, 75, 357
Doyle, M. G.	313
Dumont, T. D.	20, 95, 96
Duncanson, M. G.	108
Durney, E. C.	28, 253, 292
Dwyer, T. G.	44
Dykema, R. W.	314, 339

E

Ehrenkranz, H.	228, 244, 339
Ehrmann, E. H.	44
Eissmann, H. F.	14, 16, 17, 20, 50, 286, 313, 339
Evans, J. R.	322
Evanson, L.	205

F

Fagin, M. D.	339
Federick, D. R.	20, 123, 143, 144, 228, 244

Fellman, S.   20, 24, 34, 75
Feiglin, B.   44
Fisher, D. W.   15, 20, 33, 34, 45, 53
Fishman, I.   20, 190
Frank, A. L.   16, 143
Franklin, M. E.   228, 244, 339
Fujimoto, J.   314, 339
Fuller, J. L.   314, 339

G

Garman, T. A.   314
Gentile, D.   20, 45
George, L.   314
Gerstein, H.   28, 205
Goerig, A. C.   20, 33, 123, 292
Going, R. E.   313, 324
Goldrich, N.   123
Grant, A. A.   258
Greenberg, M.   20
Greene, G. S.   33
Greenwald, A. S.   20, 33, 79
Gruenwald, S.   205
Gutmann, J. L.   15, 20, 25, 33
Guzy, G. E.   16

H

Hamilton, A. I.   20
Hampson, E. L.   13, 19, 24, 25, 28, 163
Hannah, C. McD.   53, 357
Hanson, E. C.   19, 24, 26, 28, 29, 33, 163,
                                  241, 253
Harrington, G. W.   44
Harris, W. E.   123, 228
Harris, W. T.   20, 45
Harty, F. J.   205
Healey, H. J.   16, 20, 205
Henry, P. J.   16, 24, 28, 45, 75, 95, 96,
                         123, 143, 253, 291
Herschman, J. B.   291, 292
Hirschfeld, Z.   15, 21, 22, 24, 25, 26
Hoag, E. P.   44
Hodosh, M.   33
Holcomb, J.   275, 291
Holmlund, L.   205
Holt, J. K.   45, 357
Hormati, A. A.   314, 339
Howe, D. F.   339

J

Jacoby, W. E.   20, 45, 181
Jeannet, D. J.   34
Jensen, J. R.   314, 339
Johansson, G.   44
Johnson, J. K.   16, 19, 24, 26, 163, 181,
                 291, 292, 314, 318, 321, 339

K

Kahn, H.   20, 181, 190
Kantor, M. E.   16, 227
Kayser, A. F.   20
Kessler, J. C.   23, 30, 31
Khowassah, M. A.   314, 339
Kneller, F.   44
Kochavi, D.   255
Krejci, R. F.   44
Krupp, J. D.   19, 26, 33, 164, 241
Kurer, H. G.   228, 253, 255, 258
Kurer, P. F.   22, 228, 253, 254, 255
Kwan, E. H.   44
Kwan, S. K.   34

L

Landwerlen, J. R.   339
Larato, D. C.   20
Larson, T. D.   339
Laswell, H. R.   313, 314
Lau, V. S. M.   15, 181, 253
Leggett, L. J.   44
LeGro, A. L.   291
Lehman, M. L.   19, 24, 25, 28, 163
Leonard, L. A.   314, 316
Lerner, T. R.   314
Light, E. I.   346
Lister, A. E.   96
Lloyd, R. W.   357
Lommel, T. J.   28
Lorencki, S. F.   15, 16, 20, 253
Lovdahl, P. E.   20, 95, 96, 315
Lund, M. R.   15, 19, 28, 253

M

Malone, W. F.   20, 190
Markley, M. R.   313

Mazzuchelli, L.   24, 33, 75, 79
McLean, J. W.   75, 81
McPherson, J. L.   20, 33, 164
Messing, J. J.   258
Metrick, L.   20, 45, 53
Meyer, H. I.   44
Michnick, B. T.   75, 96, 357
Miller, A. W.   20, 22, 25, 33, 45, 53, 181
Millstein, P. L.   339
Mirman, M.   33
Mitchell, P. S.   20, 205, 211
Moffa, J. P.   313
Mohamed, S. E.   228, 244, 339
Mohammed, H.   20, 24, 143
Mondelli, J.   20, 45
Morris, D. R.   45
Morrison, K.   20, 205, 357
Moser, J.   45
Mueninghoff, L. A.   20, 33, 292
Muroff, F. I.   16, 22, 25, 95, 253, 291
Myers, A. Q.   44

N

Nathanson, D.   339
Nayyar, A.   314, 316
Neagley, R. L.   33
Neaverth, E. J.   44
Newburg, R. E.   228, 229, 230, 339
Nicholls, J. I.   16, 315
Norman, R. D.   314, 339

O

Omnell, K.-A.   292
O'Neal, R. B.   20, 228
Outhwaite, W. C.   314

P

Padgett, J. G.   123
Pameijer, C. H.   228, 229, 230, 339
Pashley, D. H.   314
Perel, M. L.   16, 22, 25, 95, 253, 291
Perez-Moll, J. F.   339
Petersen, K. B.   44
Phillips, R. W.   108, 314, 339
Piccino, A. C.   20, 45

Pickard, H. M.   20, 21
Pines, M. S.   16, 227
Pinkley, V. A.   45
Pipko, D. J.   20, 24, 205
Pokorny, M.   20
Pollack, M. H.   63, 181, 253, 258, 260, 267
Priddy, W. L.   20, 96
Priest, G.   20, 123
Prothero, J. H.   13

R

Radke, R. A.   14, 16, 17, 20, 50, 286, 313, 339
Rakow, B.   346
Ram, Z.   45, 227
Raoufi, M.   123
Raskin, R. B.   75, 96, 357
Razzano, M. R.   313
Ribbons, J. W.   44
Richardson, J. T.   123
Roane, J. B.   96
Roberts, E. W.   314
Rosen, H.   15, 20, 28, 34, 45, 53, 95, 253, 292
Rosenberg, P. A.   20, 24, 33, 45
Rosenstiel, E.   15, 75, 81
Rud, J.   292
Ruemping, D. R.   15, 19, 28, 253

S

Sabala, C. L.   16, 20
Sakumura, J. S.   19, 24, 26, 163
Sall, H. D.   15, 22, 24, 75, 79, 81
Samani, S. I. A.   20, 45
Sapone, J.   15, 16, 20, 253
Schlagel, E.   314
Schmidt, J. R.   228, 244, 339
Schnell, F. J.   33
Schnell, R. J.   15, 19, 28, 253
Schwartz, N. L.   16, 24, 26, 181, 291, 292, 314, 318, 321, 339
Scully, B. R.   44
Segat, L.   16, 20
Serene, T. P.   143, 144
Shadman, H.   22
Shaykin, J. B.   33
Sheets, C. E.   34, 205

Sherman, J. A.	227	
Shillingburg, H. T.	15, 20, 23, 30, 31, 33, 45, 53, 96	
Shirdel, K.	123	
Shulman, L. S.	339	
Sicklemore, F. A.	44	
Silness, J.	44	
Silverstein, W. H.	20, 45, 53	
Skurnik, H.	24	
Sotera, A. J.	44	
Sox, J. T.	123	
Spalten, R. G.	227, 339	
Spanauf, A. J.	228	
Spang, H.	275	
Spangler, C. C.	20, 28, 33, 95	
Stahl, G. J.	20, 228	
Standlee, J. P.	15, 19, 24, 25, 26, 27, 28, 29, 33, 63, 163, 164, 181, 240, 241, 253, 258, 260, 267, 275, 291, 292, 313, 314, 322, 344	
Steele, G. D.	228	
Stern, N.	15, 21, 22, 24, 25, 26, 45, 255	
Stovall, J.	313	
Strauss, S.	291, 292	
Svare, C. W.	339	
Symons, B.	314	

T

Tamarin, A. H.	13
Taylor, A. G.	15, 16, 20, 33, 45
Taylor, G. N.	20, 181, 190
Tebrock, O. C.	123
Thayer, K. E.	20, 24, 143

Tidmarsh, B.	16, 20, 28, 292
Tilk, M. A.	28
Trabert, K. C.	17, 19, 26, 33, 164, 241, 275

W

Waldman, P. M.	45, 357
Waliszewski, K. J.	16, 20
Walton, R. E.	314, 316
Ward, N. L.	20, 21
Warren, S. R.	44
Watson, R. J.	228, 314
Wax, A. H.	20, 181, 190
Wearn, D. I.	96
Weine, F. S.	20, 181, 190, 291, 292
Welk, D. A.	313, 314
Welsh, S. L.	20, 96
Wetz, J. H.	322
Whiteside, W. D.	228
Wictorin, L.	205
Wiland, L.	20, 45, 53, 357
Wills, D. J.	258
Wilson, E. L.	23, 30, 31
Wilson, K. R.	96
Wing, G.	313

Y

Yuodelis, R.	20, 205, 357

Z

Zak, E. L.	33
Zmener, O.	253, 257, 292

Subject Index

A

Abutment	161, 227, 318, 340
Acrylic, Duralay	56, 131, 132, 133, 170, 178
Acrylic resin	45, 58, 59, 61, 110, 123, 129, 169, 170, 192, 205, 214, 215
Alloy	
– Base metal	45
– Gold	45, 61, 108, 135, 154, 195, 205, 218
– Nickel-chrome	45, 60, 61, 63, 135, 194, 195, 205
Amalgam	
– Coronal-radicular	314
– Pin-retained	313
– Slot retention	314
Amalgam core	69, 95, 140, 227, 228, 291, 300, 303, 310, 313, 314, 315, 324, 325, 326, 327, 328, 337
Amalgam core, retention	313, 317
Anti-rotational resistance	163, 189 211, 300
Apical filling, minimum	20
Apical seal	33

B

Base metal alloy	45
BCH system	230
Buttressing effect	228

C

Calibrated Instrumentation Kit	182, 231
Canal space	163
Cast dowel	143, 315, 339
Cast dowel-core	178, 227
Cement	
– Cyano-acrylate	33
– Epoxy	33
– Filler	150, 197
– Glass ionomer	33
– Polycarboxylate	33, 299

– Vent	33, 63, 114, 137, 152, 163, 196, 219, 220, 243, 266, 277, 283
– Zinc oxide-eugenol	339, 364, 371, 374
– Zinc phosphate	33, 63, 115, 138, 139, 157, 174, 197, 219, 241, 266, 299
Cementation, dowel	28, 33
Cemented pins	313
Centrix syringe	244, 285, 307, 347
Chamber, hydraulic	137, 266, 299
Colorama Kit	182, 231
Contra-bevel	15, 54, 58, 82, 189, 212
Core	
– Amalgam	69, 95, 140, 227, 228, 291, 300, 303, 310, 313, 314, 315, 324, 325, 326, 327, 328, 337
– Composite resin	95, 123, 227, 228, 243, 244, 245, 246, 247, 249, 276, 284, 291, 300, 307, 314, 339, 340
– Definition	14
– Pattern	205, 218
– Pin-retained	16
Corrosion	292
Counter-rotational device	15
Crown, temporary	231, 340, 357
Custom dowel-core	34, 45, 61, 75, 123, 163
Cyano-acrylate cement	33

D

Dentatus Screw Post	292, 293, 294, 295, 298, 310
Diameter, root	26
Di-Lok tray	85
Dimensions, root	28
Direct custom dowel-core	45
Direct pattern	40, 178, 205
Dowel	
– Cast	143, 315, 339
– Cementation	28, 33
– Definition	14
– Diameter	25, 26, 27, 28, 46, 99, 163, 276, 292, 294, 297,
– Length	18, 19, 20, 21, 22, 24, 50, 52,

99, 164, 186, 187, 210, 236, 292, 294, 297
- Paper clip 357, 358, 359, 360, 361, 369
- Parallel 24, 28, 163, 205, 228, 275
- Parallel, self-threading 275, 278
- Plastic pattern 169, 170
- Precision plastic 123, 163, 178, 181, 195
- Prefabricated 40, 123, 143, 163, 167, 205, 206, 212, 227, 228, 238
- Prefabricated, metal 95
- Preparation 33, 164, 182, 187, 205, 209, 237, 280, 297
- Reinforcement by 16
- Secondary intention 143
- Serrated 28, 163, 205, 230, 232, 253, 275
- Serrated, parallel plastic 163
- Smooth-sided 28
- Space 127, 148, 163, 166, 177, 237, 256, 280, 297
- Spring-loaded 13
- Stainless steel 227, 228, 231, 232, 241, 249, 275, 292
- Surface 28
- Taper 24, 28, 181, 182, 291
- Tapered 163, 181, 183, 184, 190, 195, 205, 206, 228, 231, 291
- Tapered, threaded 140, 291, 295
- Tapered, plastic 181, 190, 195
- Threaded 28, 140, 228, 253, 275, 291, 295
- Wrought 205
Dowel-core 14, 16
- Cast 178, 227
- Custom 34, 45, 61, 75, 123, 163
- Multiple piece 95
- Para-Post 165
- Pattern 55, 61, 68, 70, 71, 123, 135, 141, 172, 195, 201
- Posterior 66, 95
- Preparation 55, 184, 207, 233, 278
- Two-piece 95, 227, 318
Dowel-crown 357
Dowel-inlay 143, 144, 155, 156, 159, 160, 162, 228
Dowel-inlay pattern 149, 153
Drills
- Gates Glidden 33, 34, 148, 236
- Paramax 164
- Para-Post 164, 166, 177, 229, 237
Duralay acrylic 56, 131, 132, 133, 170, 178

E
Endodontic files 187, 200, 205, 206, 209
Endopost 205, 206, 222, 224
Endowel 183, 190, 201, 202
Engine reamers 182, 183, 256
Epoxy cement 33

F
Ferrule effect 14, 50, 228
Files, endodontic 187, 200, 205, 206, 209
Fracture, root 21, 26, 28, 292

G
Gates Glidden drills 33, 34, 148, 236
Glass ionomer cement 33
Gold alloy 45, 61, 108, 135, 154, 195, 205, 218
Gutta percha 33, 34, 177
Gypsum-bonded investment 135, 154, 195, 218

H
Hydraulic chamber 137, 266, 299

I
Impression 75, 83, 85, 101, 103, 149, 150, 164, 190, 214
Indirect fabrication 40, 149, 164, 190, 205
Inlay 143
Investment
- Gypsum-bonded 135, 154
- Phosphate-bonded 135, 195
Iridio-platinum pins 164

K
Keyway 15, 45, 53, 61, 81, 120, 121, 122, 128, 129, 164, 170, 189, 211
Kurer posts 228, 253, 254, 270
Kurer reamer 254, 257, 270

L

Lateral stress 137, 219
Lentulo spiral 63, 75, 84, 102, 115, 138,
150, 157, 174, 197, 220,
241, 283, 299

M

Maillefer reamer 276, 280
Mallet 64, 116

N

Nickel-chrome alloy 45, 135, 194, 195, 205
Non-rigid connector 95, 119
NuBond Fast Post 232

P

Parallel
– Dowel 24, 28, 163, 175, 205, 228
– Pins 15, 163, 164, 167, 168, 178
– Self-threading dowel 275, 278
– Threaded dowel 253, 255, 275
Paralleling jig 164, 167, 168
Paramax twist drill 164, 167, 168, 178
Para-Post 163, 165, 172, 178, 232, 242, 250
Para-Post drill 164, 166, 177, 229, 237
Paste filler 138, 157
Pattern
– Dowel-core 123, 135, 141, 172, 195, 201
– Dowel-inlay 149, 153
– Direct 40, 178, 205
– Indirect 40
– Prefabricated precision 45, 75
– Wax 152, 154, 161, 164
P-D posts 183, 232
Peeso reamer 33, 34, 45, 51, 56, 77, 80,
99, 127, 148, 166, 188, 229,
236, 237, 254, 257, 275, 280,
293, 294
Perforation 25, 27, 181, 321
Phosphate-bonded investment 135, 195
Pins 228, 238–240, 314, 315, 316, 317
– Cemented 313
– Iridio-platinum 164, 169, 170
– Parallel 15, 163, 164, 167, 168, 178
– Placement 321–324, 343–345
– Plastic 164

– Self-threading 313
Pin-retained amalgam 313
Pin-retained core 16
Pin-temporary crown 357, 358, 359, 360,
361, 362, 363, 364,
365, 369, 370, 371
Pivot crown 13
Plastic
– Dowel pattern 169, 170
– Pins 164
– Posts 164
– Shell 357, 367, 368, 369
– Sprues 54, 104, 110, 129, 130
Polycarbonate crown 357, 358, 361, 363
Polycarboxylate cement 33, 299
Post 14
Post, plastic 164
Precision attachment 121
Precision plastic dowel 123, 163, 178,
181, 195
Prefabricated dowel 40, 123, 143, 163,
167, 205, 206, 212,
227, 228, 238
Prefabricated precision pattern 45, 75
Prefabricated metal dowel 95
Preparation, dowel 33, 164, 182, 187,
205, 209, 280, 297
Principle of Substitution 13
Pulp cap 143

R

Radix anchor 275, 276, 277, 287, 288
Reamer 181, 205
– Engine 182, 183, 256
– Kurer 254, 257, 270
– Maillefer 276, 280
– Peeso 33, 34, 45, 51, 56, 77, 80, 99,
127, 148, 166, 188, 229, 236,
237, 254, 257, 275, 280, 293, 294
Resistance 143, 163, 227, 228, 230, 275,
315, 339
Retention 18, 24, 26, 28, 143, 163, 164,
229, 253, 275, 291, 339
Retention, amalgam core 313, 317
Richmond crown 13
Root
– Diameter 26
– Dimensions 28
– Facer 254, 258, 270

– Fracture 21, 26, 28, 292
– Splitting 24, 25

S

Secondary intention dowel 143
Self-threading pins 313
Serrated dowel 28, 163, 205, 230,
232, 253, 275
Serrated surface 163, 230, 232
Shell, custom plastic 357, 367, 368, 369
Silver point 33, 123, 177
Slot retention, amalgam 314
Smooth-sided dowel 28
Splitting forces 228
Sprue, plastic 57, 104, 110, 129, 130
Stainless steel dowel 227, 228, 231, 232,
241, 249, 275, 292
Stress 137, 181, 219, 253, 267, 275, 291
Stress, lateral 137, 219
Surface, dowel 28
Surface, serrated 163, 230, 232
Syringe, Centrix 244, 285, 307, 347

T

Taper, dowel 24, 28, 181, 182, 291
Tapered dowel 163, 181, 184, 205, 206,
228, 231, 291

Tapered threaded dowel 140, 291, 295
Temporary crown 231, 340, 357
Temporary crown, acrylic 357, 361, 370
Threaded dowel 28, 140, 228, 253, 275,
291, 295

V

Vent, cement 33, 63, 114, 137, 152, 163,
196, 219, 220, 243, 266, 277, 283

W

Wax forms 87, 105
Wax pattern 86, 88, 89, 104, 152, 154,
161, 164
Wedging effect 181, 291

Z

Zinc oxide-eugenol cement 339, 364,
371, 374
Zinc phosphate cement 33, 63, 115, 138,
139, 157, 174, 197,
219, 241, 266, 299

quintessence
books

Dean L. Johnson/Russel J. Stratton

Fundamentals of
Removable Prosthodontics

To achieve the greatest benefit from prosthodontic treatment, the principles of prevention must become an integral part of diagnosis.

The philosophy of partial denture treatment described here includes patient motivation toward maintenance of oral hygiene, mouth preparation, appropriate distribution of functional stress, selection of the cleanest designs, exclusion of unnecessary elements, and striving to avoid complete edentulousness for the patient.

ISBN 0-931386-10-1

504 pages, 458 illustrations, size 17.5 × 24.5 cm,
linen bound with gold stamping and protective cover.
Quintessence Publishing Co. Inc.
8 South Michigan Avenue, Suite 2301 · Chicago, Illinois 60603

quintessence
books

Shillingburg/Wilson/Morrison

Guide to Occlusal Waxing

To reinforce the lessons taught by the study of dental morphology, to help put into practice the knowledge of occlusal form and function, this manual leads the reader through the steps of occlusal waxing.

Every step, and every procedure is illustrated with stylized drawings. Groove and ridge patterns, location of occlusal contacts, and excursion paths traced by opposing cusp tips are developed to aid the student in making the transition from novice to expert.

The drawings and their legends alone offer a wealth of information.

ISBN 0-931386-03-9

45 pages, 125 illustrations (46 in color)
size 17 × 24 cm, spiralbound
Quintessence Publishing Co. Inc.
8 South Michigan Avenue, Suite 2301 · Chicago, Illinois 60603